Preparation for the Praxis

in Speech-Language Pathology

Preparation for the Praxis
in Speech-Language Pathology

Kay T. Payne

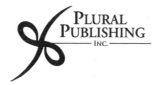
PLURAL
PUBLISHING
INC.

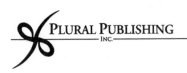

5521 Ruffin Road
San Diego, CA 92123

Email: information@pluralpublishing.com
Website: https://www.pluralpublishing.com

Typeset in 12/14 Adobe Garamond by Flanagan's Publishing Services, Inc.
Printed in the United States of America by Integrated Books International

Library of Congress Cataloging-in-Publication Data:

Names: Payne, Kay T., author.
Title: Preparation for the Praxis in speech-language pathology / Kay T. Payne.
Description: San Diego, CA : Plural Publishing, Inc., [2020] | Includes
    bibliographical references and index.
Identifiers: LCCN 2019053127 | ISBN 9781635503142 (paperback) | ISBN
    9781635503197 (ebook)
Subjects: MESH: Speech Disorders | Language Disorders | Examination
    Question | Study Guide
Classification: LCC RC424.7 | NLM WV 18.2 | DDC 616.85/5—dc23
LC record available at https://lccn.loc.gov/2019053127

Contents

Preface

Congratulations! You have selected the most comprehensive and in-depth resource for preparing for the Speech-Language Pathology Praxis. *Preparation for the Praxis in Speech-Language Pathology* is so much more than the conventional review manual as its focus is on you, the test taker, rather than the test content. This volume provides mental preparation in everyday language, speaking directly to the reader to break the mystique surrounding the Praxis and develop usable skills for optimizing performance.

Inside you will discover discussion on studying for the Praxis, misconceptions and facts, cognitive abilities, reasoning skills, reading comprehension, mental preparation, test-taking strategy, time utilization, and guessing strategies. Each instructional chapter presents enlightening information accompanied by demonstrative examples to give the reader valuable practice with Praxis-type questions, plus real frequently asked questions gathered from students' queries over many years. Also included are stimulating personal exercises to assess your level of preparedness such as study habits, test anxiety, reading speed, and reading comprehension.

Assess your academic knowledge, strengths, and weaknesses using the 19 coursework quizzes from both undergraduate prerequisites and graduate courses. A full Coursework Study Guide lists what to study in each Praxis content area and demonstrates through actual Praxis questions, listed in the references as "Sources," how concrete knowledge must be applied for clinical decisions, as well as the use of relevant reasoning skills.

To complete the experience, a full-length timed Praxis Practice Test allows you to hone the acquired skills gained through the instructional chapters and gain valuable practice. Detailed explanations to correct, as well as incorrect, answers teach you to think like the item-writer and reason as the writer intended.

Whether you are a verdant student or a seasoned professional returning to the field, you will find this amazing resource essential as you prepare for the Speech-Language Pathology Praxis.

Chapter 1

Study Habits

Before you sit down to study for an exam as important as the Praxis, you should consider your study habits, as well as what is required to successfully complete the exam. Begin with the following study habits exercise. Record your answers on a separate sheet, tally your results according to the key presented, and note the interpretation of your score.

Study Habits Questionnaire

1. How would you describe your usual study habits in relation to your testing success?
   A. I don't have to study much to get good grades
   B. The more I study, the better my grades
   C. If I don't study, my grades suffer
   D. Even when I study more, my grades are just about the same

2. How often do you feel that you have studied, but the exam focused on other information?
   A. Never
   B. Rarely
   C. Sometimes
   D. Often

3. How often do you misjudge what is to be included on an exam? That is, do you ever avoid studying some material and take a chance that it will not be on the exam, but it does appear on the exam?
   A. Never
   B. Rarely
   C. Sometimes
   D. Often

4. How often do you find that you have studied as much as or more than your peers, but your grades are not as high?
   A. Never
   B. Rarely
   C. Sometimes
   D. Often

5. On what kind of question do you perform best?
   A. Multiple Choice
   B. Fill-In/True-False
   C. Matching
   D. Essay

6. On what kind of question do you perform worst?
   A. There is no difference
   B. Essay
   C. True-False/Matching/Fill-In
   D. Multiple Choice

7. When you guess on a question, how often are you correct?
   A. Often
   B. Sometimes
   C. Rarely
   D. Never

8. How often do you observe that you have misinterpreted a question?
   A. Never
   B. Rarely
   C. Sometimes
   D. Often

9. How often do you feel that you know more than your exam scores reflect?
   A. Never
   B. Rarely
   C. Sometimes
   D. Often

10. Are your scores on standardized tests consistent with your academic grades?
    A. Standardized test scores are higher than grades
    B. Grades and standardized test scores are consistent

C. Standardized test scores are somewhat lower than grades

D. Standardized test scores are definitely lower than grades

A = 4

B = 3

C = 2

D = 1

26–30 Points: **Excellent**

Your study habits are conducive to good performance. You probably learn very well in class; thus, extensive study time may not be required. Your intuitive skills for predicting what will be on the exam are also quite good. You are probably a good test taker regardless of the type of question.

21–25 Points: **Above Average**

Your study skills are adequate. You probably perform well despite a few qualities that are less than optimal. Note the consistency of your responses; e.g., whether they lie in amount of study time, types of questions, or judgment of the content of the exam. With this knowledge you can improve the quality of your study experience.

16–20 Points: **Average**

You often selected "C" as your answer. Although you may know the course content, you are an average to below-average test taker. Be acutely aware that effective studying is a matter of *process* as well content and time. Practicing the types of questions that will appear on the Praxis is the most effective study process. In addition, it is helpful to know and understand as much about the Praxis as possible. Read all information about the Praxis presented in the bulletin that is available on the Educational Testing Service (ETS) website. In addition, you must tailor your studying not only to the specific content areas of the exam, but also to your individual strengths and weaknesses, whether in the subject areas, amount of time, study procedures, or the types of questions. If you are usually wrong when you guess, you must improve your intuitive ability. Your study should be designed to compensate for your personal weaknesses.

Less than 20 Points: **Below Average**

You are at high risk for poor performance on the Praxis. Bear in mind that you may know the course information well, but for some reason your test performance is not good, or that you may need to review the course information. Read all information about the Praxis presented on the Educational Testing Service (ETS) website. In addition, you must tailor your studying not only to the specific content areas of the exam, but also to your individual strengths and weaknesses, whether in the subject areas, amount of time, study procedures, or the types of questions. If you are usually wrong when you guess on an exam, you must improve your intuitive ability. Your studying should be designed to compensate for your personal weaknesses. If you are not adept at taking multiple-choice tests, perhaps the reason relates to your decision-making ability.

Often the presence of more than one plausible response creates confusion. To lessen this confusion, use your internal powers of concentration, reasoning, and confidence. These powers can be perfected with extensive practice with Praxis-type questions.

What to Study

Effective studying is more a matter of process than of content or volume. Yet some review of coursework will be necessary. Review of coursework is especially recommended if you completed your academic study more than 1 year prior to taking the Praxis. While many Praxis questions require verbatim recall of information, most questions are presented as clinical scenarios for which a broad understanding of each course is necessary.

It is important to note, however, that performance is enhanced more by intuitive skills of *clinical judgment, critical thinking, test-taking strategy, timing,* and *effective guessing.* In some cases, good test takers—i.e., those who are able to utilize these five skills—sometimes perform well even without course knowledge. However, for most examinees it is a wise choice to practice the requisite skills, as well as to have knowledge of the field.

Many individuals presume they should study their weakest areas or the most difficult courses. These strategies are **not** recommended in preparation for the Praxis for two reasons. First, there may be no more than five or six questions from any specific course area. Therefore, it is conceivable to pass the Praxis even if you have not taken some courses.

Second, questions from courses that are sometimes most difficult (e.g., anatomy) are not presented for specific recall of information. Instead, a question may examine your knowledge of anatomy in the context of a clinical example. Thus, it is necessary to know anatomy as it relates to specific disorders, as in the following sample question.

Which of the following is the most significant contributor to impairment in the speech of persons with an unrepaired cleft palate?

    A. Irregular vocal fold function

    B. Hearing loss from otitis media

    C. Velopharyngeal insufficiency

    D. Persistent faulty articulatory patterns

(C) The most common speech impairment of persons with cleft palate is hypernasality. Velopharyngeal insufficiency is the main factor contributing to hypernasality, therefore the correct answer is (C). (A) is incorrect because vocal fold function is not associated with cleft palate. (B) is incorrect because otitis media is not always present with cleft palate. (D) is incorrect because faulty articulatory patterns are subject to compensatory strategies.

Some required courses, such as statistics, are not examined directly. Hence, they should be reviewed broadly, but not emphasized for extended study.

In addition, the Praxis will contain questions in knowledge of areas in which you may not have had a specific course. The list below contains areas that are included and strongly recommended for emphasis as you review.

■ Multicultural Issues

■ Speech Science

■ Language Development

■ Ethics/Professional Issues

■ Phonetics

■ Linguistics

■ Counseling

How to Study

■ Become familiar with all the content areas of the exam. You may need to study some areas more than others. However, you should determine how much time to devote to each area based on the number of questions, as well as your estimation of the difficulty of the content areas and the amount of knowledge you have in each area.

■ GET ORGANIZED! Begin to study at least 2 or 3 months prior to the exam date. Plan a schedule of which areas you will study each week. Adopt a regular and realistic study routine. Set aside a block of hours per week for study.

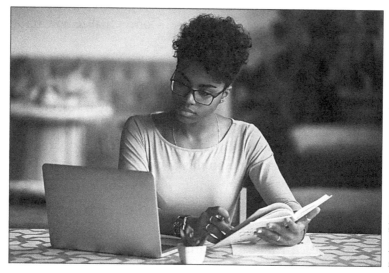

iStock.com/fizkes

Discipline yourself to keep to your study routine. If you miss study hours, make them up at another time.

■ Maintain a daily study log showing the dates, times, and subjects you study. This will help to chart your progress, pace yourself, and note areas remaining to be reviewed. Jot down on index cards the specific points you wish to refresh before the exam.

■ Review both graduate and undergraduate coursework.

■ Review class notes, retake old exams, and look at textbooks other than the ones used in your classes. Memorize important facts, but also seek to understand and integrate the material so that it will be thoroughly comprehended and retained.

■ If you are studying for your master's comprehensive, remember that the Praxis will cover material from undergraduate courses not included on your comprehensive exam. In addition, the knowledge required for the Praxis may be more general in nature. Therefore, you may need to tailor your study strategies to meet the demands of the Praxis.

■ Know the areas of the Praxis for which you may not have had specific coursework. Become familiar with the information in these areas.

■ Form study groups of at least two other people. Exchange notes with other students, especially those from other universities, through social media. Make your own difficult questions within the study group and quiz each other. Discuss the answers.

■ If you have been away from coursework for an extended time, a review course, self-study workshop, or review textbook may be required. You may also select a comprehensive introductory textbook to review. Textbooks with accompanying multiple-choice study questions are most helpful. Even if you attend a review course, an introductory text is advisable.

■ Although some factual information is necessary, don't study to memorize facts. Instead, study to update your knowledge. Conceptualize how information can be used in a clinical example.

■ Don't put more emphasis on the subjects that were difficult for you. Rather, emphasize the areas of coursework you may be lacking.

■ PRACTICE. PRACTICE. PRACTICE. Particularly if you are not a good test taker. Seek as many opportunities for practice with Praxis-type questions as possible. Practice to increase your timing and reading speed, as well as to increase the skills and strategies in this book. Retake the exam at a later time and compare results.

The ETS Praxis website provides information about the content of the Praxis and study tips. Specific information about the Praxis registration and content is also available from the American Speech-Language-Hearing Association (ASHA) website.

Chapter 2

Misconceptions and Facts

Gathering knowledge and information about the exam is an effective study strategy. Since standardized tests such as the Praxis are unlike the classroom exams with which you are most familiar, it is of utmost importance to have a thorough understanding of the nature of standardized tests to maximize your performance.

A standardized test is one in which performance scores of each individual examinee are compared with the mean for all others who took the exam at the same time. For the Praxis, there is one cut score, but with each administration the number of correct answers needed to reach the passing mark varies. Thus, the number of correct answers needed to pass the Praxis may differ upward or downward depending on when the exam is taken. Before you complete this chapter, test your knowledge with the following quiz.

What Do I Know About the Praxis?

1. There are 150 questions on the Praxis.
   A. True   B. False

2. There are four answer choices for all Praxis questions.
   A. True   B. False

3. If you don't know the answer, you should leave it blank.
   A. True   B. False

4. You have two hours to take the Praxis.
   A. True   B. False

5. The passing score for the Praxis is 162.
   A. True   B. False

6. You must pass the Praxis before your clinical fellowship year.
   A. True   B. False

7. You can only take the Praxis two times.

   A. True   B. False

8. The Praxis is given online.

   A. True   B. False

9. The Praxis covers the master's curriculum only.

   A. True   B. False

10. Scores on the Praxis are active for 10 years.

    A. True   B. False

Answers

1. (B) *False* There are 132 multiple choice questions on the Praxis.

2. (A) *True* Each question has four answer choices.

3. (B) *False* You should always fill in an answer; however, there are ways to improve your guessing ability, which will be discussed in a future chapter.

4. (B) *False* You are given 2.5 hours to take the Praxis.

5. (A) *True* The passing score is 162; however, this may be different for state licensure and other purposes of the Praxis.

6. (B) *False* For optimal performance it is recommended that you take the Praxis before the clinical fellowship year, but it is not a requirement.

7. (B) *False* There is no limit to the number of times you can take the Praxis. If you apply to the American Speech-Language-Hearing Association (ASHA) for certification, you can submit scores from two Praxis exams. If you require more than two times, you will need to submit another application to ASHA.

8. (A) *True* The Praxis is an online test.

9. (B) *False* The Praxis will contain questions from undergraduate courses such as language development, phonetics, and aural rehabilitation.

10. (B) *False* Educational Testing Service (ETS) will retain your scores for 10 years. However, ASHA requires a score within the previous 5 years.

Scoring

Calculate the percentage of correct answers. Whatever your score, whether high or low, you should read all available information about the Praxis. Do not depend on hearsay for your information. Become aware and do not be influenced by the misconceptions and myths you may have heard from others.

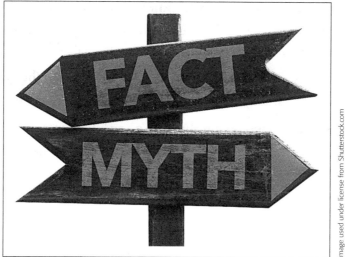

Misconceptions

Traditionally, there have been many rumors and misconceptions resulting from lack of knowledge and understanding of standardized tests. The greatest danger of these misconceptions is that they contribute to test anxiety, which has the possibility of diminishing performance. The effect of misconceptions can be so strong that, even in the face of evidence to the contrary, some examinees cling persistently to the falsehoods, and thus create unnecessary and often deleterious coping mechanisms.

A list of common misconceptions about the Praxis is presented below, followed by a list of facts. The list of misconceptions could probably be expanded indefinitely. The best advice to examinees is to read all information about the test, and distrust any accounts that are inconsistent with the written information.

■ **The best time to take the Praxis is after the clinical fellowship year.**

The optimal time to take the Praxis is near the end of your master's program. Students in training receive higher scores than other individuals because the Praxis is created for students and recent graduates.

■ **You cannot study for the Praxis.**

Some questions on the Praxis require recall of specific subject matter. However, it is best to practice to improve your test-taking skills.

■ **The Praxis is an online exam.**

The Praxis is given online with an appointment at an approved testing center.

■ **You can only take the Praxis two times.**

Neither ASHA nor ETS restrict the number of times that the Praxis may be taken.

■ **If you are not sure of an answer, skip it and leave it blank.**

Only correct answers are scored. Skipped questions are scored as wrong answers. There is no penalty for wrong answers. Effective guessing is a valuable test-taking strategy.

■ **You don't have to answer more than (some fraction) of the questions to pass.**

Strive to answer all questions to increase your performance. Don't skip any answers.

■ **The Praxis always has an emphasis (e.g., swallowing, stuttering).**

A set number of questions is assigned to each of three content areas. No area is disproportionally represented.

■ **The Praxis focuses only on master's-level study.**

The scope of the Praxis includes both undergraduate and master's study.

■ **You cannot take the Praxis if you don't have a master's degree.**

The Praxis is used by organizations for various purposes. It is sometimes taken by those without a master's degree, especially students in their master's program.

■ **You must report your score to ASHA every time you take the Praxis.**

When you register for the Praxis you may select to have the scores sent to you or to any institution you designate. Scores are sent only to the institutions you designate. Score reports requested after registration incur an additional fee. You may also cancel your score report designations before they are sent.

■ **Every version of the Praxis has a whole new set of questions.**

Some questions may be repeated from previous versions of the Praxis.

■ **Some schools have the Praxis to pass out to their students prior to the exam.**

The Praxis is security protected and is not available for early distribution.

■ **If you don't pass the Praxis, you cannot get a job in the field.**

While most jobs require ASHA certification or state licensure, it is possible to work in the field without passing the Praxis, especially during the clinical fellowship year.

■ **My classmate has better grades and she did not pass. That means I won't pass either.**

Some examinees are poor test takers even though they have knowledge of the material. It is not possible to judge your performance by someone else.

Facts

- There are 132 questions on the Praxis.
- You are given 2.5 hours to complete the exam.
- You have less than 1 minute per question.

- All questions are multiple choice.

- All questions have four answer choices.

- No points are subtracted from your total correct responses as a penalty for guessing.

- You will need a score of 162 to pass the exam.

- You can pass the Praxis by correctly answering about 60% to 65% of the questions.

- The Praxis exam covers both your undergraduate and graduate study.

- Based on the percentage of questions answered correctly by examinees, the most difficult questions for speech-language pathology are in neurogenic disorders and basic human communication processes.

- Most questions on the Praxis are not recall questions. You may be given an example or a clinical scenario and asked to make judgments, identify, classify, or interpret information.

- The Praxis may contain charts, graphs, spectrograms, audiograms, and tympanograms that you will be required to analyze and interpret.

- Many questions on the Praxis will require you to make clinical judgments or use common sense.

Frequently Asked Questions

- I find it difficult to select the textbook answer in a case scenario question. How do you avoid applying your clinical experience? I would think those experiences would be beneficial for the Praxis.

The textbook response refers to the "generally accepted" response. In your personal clinical experience, you have dealt with complex individual cases. Probably few have been "textbook" examples. The Praxis is designed to reflect the common knowledge of the field, not individual personal experiences.

- I heard that when guessing, one should mark the same answer for all the questions. Is there a letter that works most often? Or should I just randomly choose a letter and stick with it?

Your question reflects a popular myth. In fact, choosing "C" (for example) for every guess probably won't improve your score by very much. In a future chapter we will discuss the difference between random guessing and educated guessing.

- Why is skipping around not recommended? I find that I have more confidence if I skip to questions where I am confident in my answer choice.

If this is a coping strategy that relieves test anxiety and works for you, then it is fine. As a general rule, it is probably not feasible for every examinee.

- You shared that the Praxis requires test-taking skills rather than memory. Other than practice tests, how should I practice test-taking skills?

After taking the practice test, read the explanations for the answers you missed gleaning the implied logic. Retake the test employing similar logic.

- It was stated that there is less than a minute per question. I was under the impression that I have more than a minute. How can I skim questions to avoid wasting time?

Don't plan to utilize more than 1 minute per question. Some questions require as little as 10 seconds, and some will require more than a minute. Skimming is not recommended. Future chapters will discuss timing and reading speed.

- One myth is that you cannot study for the exam. Aren't there recall questions on general information? Why isn't it best to review the basics in each subject area?

There will be several recall questions, but most questions will require critical thinking and clinical judgment. These skills are perfected through experience and practice with Praxis-type questions.

- I've known people who passed the Praxis without any graduate work. Is it really important to put a lot of emphasis on studying?

Some exceptional individuals are very good test takers who use strategies well with a limited amount of information. It is important to know your personal strengths and weaknesses and study to accommodate any weaknesses.

- I notice that a lot of questions were from undergraduate courses. I do not recall much of that information, and I also have weaknesses in graduate courses. What should I focus on so that I do not get overwhelmed with too much information?

It is important to organize your study to incorporate each of the test areas, focusing on weaknesses but not excluding essential courses.

- When the Praxis is given will everyone receive the same questions?

Each test administration is individualized. However, you may find some questions repeated from a previous time.

- How is the room set up for the Praxis? Are we stuffed into one room and constantly monitored, or will we have quiet and elbow room?

The test environment will be comfortable, appropriate, and monitored. Depending on the test center to which you are assigned, there may be others who are taking a different test.

- Since the Praxis can be taken before the clinical fellowship year, has research shown that individuals tend to score lower if they wait to take the test after the clinical fellowship year?

The Praxis is designed for students and recent graduates. It is logical that the more recently you completed your graduate study, the better your performance.

Sources

Educational Testing Service. (2011). *Extended test time for test takers whose Primary Language is Not English* (PLNE). Retrieved from http://www.ets.org/praxis/register/accommodations/plne

Educational Testing Service. (2011). *Resources for test takers with disabilities and health-related needs.* Retrieved from http://www.ets.org/disabilities

Chapter 3

Critical Thinking Skills

We have all observed how some people do well on examinations without ever seeming to study, while others study extensively without similar success. This phenomenon is perhaps due to the fact that some examinations are constructed to measure "cognitive abilities" in addition to knowledge. On these examinations, the questions require the use of specific higher-order cognitive processes to demonstrate, rather than recall, the required knowledge. These are otherwise known as *critical thinking skills*.

Generally, examinations that only test knowledge are perceived by students to be easier than examinations that require critical thinking. One possible explanation of this is that studying can enhance one's knowledge, but no amount of studying can improve intuitive cognitive abilities. Much like skillful piano playing, these abilities are developed through practice and experience.

Critical thinking involves use of higher-order thought processes that allow humans to use basic knowledge in a creative fashion. Note the difference between the following two questions as examples. The first requires basic knowledge, while the second requires critical thinking.

I. Which of the following is a phonological feature of African-American English?
   A. f/θ, initial position
   B. f/θ, medial position
   C. -/θ, final position
   D. s/θ, final position

II. Which of the following would be considered an error rather than a normal phonological process for a 6-year-old boy who speaks African-American English?
   A. [pɛn] → [hɛn]
   B. [pɛn] → [pĩ]
   C. [pɛn] → [pɛ:]
   D. [pɛn] → [pɪn]

The first question requires knowledge and recall of information. The examinee must recognize the single correct answer among the other options. This type of question is known as a *verbatim recall question.*

Note that the second question not only requires knowledge, but also application of that knowledge in a clinical example. The process of extrapolation typified by this example is an important cognitive skill for the Praxis.

Answer I

(B) A prominent feature of African-American English (AAE) is f/θ in both medial and final positions as in "baftub"/"bathtub" and "toof"/"tooth" so (B) is the correct answer. A typical speaker of AAE would not produce f/θ in initial position as in "fink"/"think" (A); or delete final /θ/ as in "o" for "oath" (C); or substitute s/θ in final position as in "bas"/"bath" (D) so these are incorrect.

Answer II

(A) Substitution of consonants (e.g., /h/ for /p/) is a true phonological error. Normal features of AAE include vowel nasalization before final nasal consonant (B); vowel extension before final nasal consonant (C); and substitution of ɪ/ɛ before a nasal consonant (D).

Cognitive Skills for the Praxis

The cognitive skills required for the Praxis are based on *Bloom's Taxonomy of Educational Objectives: Cognitive Domain* (Bloom, 1957), which are as follows:

Comprehension

Comprehension entails grasping the meaning of material, converting ideas from one form to another, explaining or summarizing material, and extending the meaning beyond data. Examples of comprehension include:

- extracting the intended theme from a verbal or written description;
- identifying and classifying a theme from a verbal or written description;
- translating examples into concepts;
- identifying research examples as a type of design; and
- identifying a hypothesis or statistical method from an example.

Application

Application involves using abstractions in either general or concrete situations. Examples of application include:

- making clinical judgments;

- making a prognosis for recovery; and
- naming a clinical problem given its characteristics.

Analysis

In analysis, the examinee breaks down material into its parts, identifies the parts, identifies the relationship among the parts, and identifies the way parts are organized. Examples of analysis include:

- finding commonalities among items such as phonemes, then suggesting a treatment strategy;
- identifying the site of lesion by speech or hearing characteristics; and
- identifying a muscle given a description of its action.

Synthesis

Synthesis is the inverse of analysis. Synthesis involves putting parts together to form a whole, a production of a unique communication, a production of a plan, a proposed set of operations, or a derivation of a set of abstract relations. Examples of synthesis include:

- selecting the best course of action in a clinical example;
- relating a type of treatment to a diagnosis and predicting possible outcomes; and
- interpreting and summarizing research results presented in tabular or graphic form.

The cognitive abilities of Bloom's taxonomy are organized hierarchically in complexity of the skills. This hierarchical order corresponds to the perceived difficulty of the questions on the Praxis. That is, the higher the cognitive required ability, the greater difficulty of the questions. Figure 3–1 depicts Bloom's taxonomical hierarchy and the difficulty level of Praxis questions that require each of the abilities.

The most difficult questions are those that require multiple cognitive abilities that must be carried out in rapid succession. Because errors of mental skill can occur at any level, correctly answering these questions demands a perfectly orchestrated process. Practicing the abilities will increase the necessary skill, thus decreasing your perception of difficulty of the questions.

Recall Questions

Recall questions require knowledge of basic information from courses. It is inevitable that questions of this type will appear on the Praxis. However, one should not expect the examination to be comprised largely of these questions. Studying and memorizing facts will enable you to correctly answer recall questions. But you can never memorize all the facts of the profession, and there is a great probability that only a few of the facts

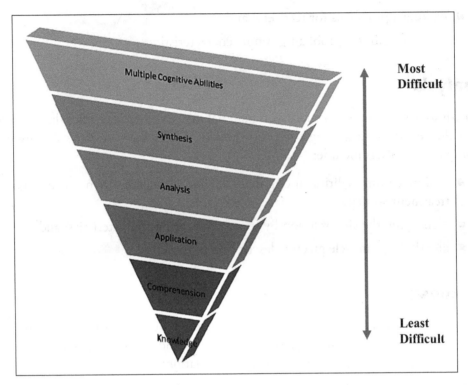

FIGURE 3–1. Question difficulty according to Bloom's taxonomical hierarchy.

you remember will appear as questions. Therefore, your rote memorization of facts should be complemented with practice with Praxis-type questions.

One advantage of recall questions is that often they can be easily answered by guessing. Even if you do not recall each fact specifically, you probably remember related information that will allow you to make an educated guess by the process of elimination. Test your knowledge or make an educated guess in the following recall question.

Which of the following qualities would a nasometer provide the most accurate information for?

A. Breathiness

B. Hyponasality

C. Hoarseness

D. Stridency

(B) A nasometer is a device for measuring nasal emission, that is, hypernasality or hyponasality. Thus, the correct answer is (B). Breathiness (A), hoarseness (C), and stridency (D) are qualities of voice production, which are not measured by a nasometer, so these are incorrect.

If you recall the information from your courses, you might immediately recognize the answer. You probably feel this was an easy question. However, let's pretend the answer was not immediately apparent. You could reason, merely by its name, that a nasometer is a measuring device for nasal activity. If you are not certain that (B) is the answer, you may work through the process of elimination with the other choices. (A), (C), and (D) would be eliminated because breathiness, hoarseness, and stridency occur at the level of the vocal folds. The next question is another example of a recall question.

Atrophic changes to which of the following is most likely to result in Huntington's chorea?

    A. Frontal lobe

    B. Cerebellum

    C. Cranial nerves

    D. Basal ganglia

(D) Huntington's chorea is a genetic disorder that leads to damage to the basal ganglia, an area of the brain with a major role in movement and behavior control. Damage results in involuntary movements and progressive dementia; therefore, the correct answer is (D). While other brain structures (A), (B), and (C) may affect muscle movement and cognitive function, these are incorrect.

    The following are Praxis-type questions requiring each of the cognitive abilities. You do not need to study or commit this information to memory. This discussion is intended to familiarize you with Praxis-type questions and their levels of difficulty. It is more important to be able to feel how each type of question becomes more difficult according to the specific cognitive demand.

Comprehension Questions

Comprehension questions often present information related to the correct answer such as a complex of symptoms. The examinee must comprehend how the information relates to the correct answer choice. Often, questions that require comprehension are distinguished visibly by their length. A typical comprehension question is wordy and contains information for the examinee to read and interpret.

A 50-year-old teacher has been referred to a speech-language pathologist by her otolaryngologist. Results of indirect laryngoscopy revealed a slight bowing of the membranous portion of the vocal folds with vocal fold edema. The teacher reports that gradually for the past 6 weeks she has experienced increased hoarseness and lower pitch that advances throughout the day as she uses her voice. Given these symptoms, the patient most likely exhibits:

    A. Contact ulcer

    B. Vocal nodule

    C. Laryngitis

    D. Myasthenia laryngis

(D) The symptoms describe the condition known as myasthenia laryngis, which is a bowing of the vocal folds, so (D) is correct. In laryngitis (C), the tissues are inflamed. Contact ulcers (A) and nodules (B) are tissue growths, so these answers are incorrect. Note how the next question requires comprehension.

Which counseling technique is reflected in the following exchange between a client's parent and a speech-language pathologist?

> *Parent:* I don't know what to do. My son is stuttering and nothing seems to help. My husband just ignores the problem.

> *Clinician:* My child is dysfluent too. I remind myself that dysfluency is sometimes a normal part of language development and he will probably grow out of it. Let's talk about how I can help your son.

A. Confrontation

B. Interpretation

C. Reflection

D. Paraphrasing

(C) In the counseling technique of reflection, the counselor offers thoughtful expansions that validate the client's feelings, so (C) is the correct answer. Reflection differs from interpretation (B) because it presents the opinion of the counselor. Reflection differs from paraphrasing (D) because reflection adds insight. Therefore (B) and (D) are incorrect. Confrontation is designed to expose hidden elements in the client's reality so (A) is also incorrect.

Application Questions

Application refers to the use of abstractions in both general and concrete situations. Examinees are often called upon to apply diagnostic and treatment principles to clinical situations, as in the following example.

A 12-year-old girl with no history of palatal cleft demonstrates nasal escape and reduced intraoral pressure on fricatives and plosive sounds. Which of the following should be given top priority in clinical management?

A. Exercises to improve velopharyngeal valving

B. Referral to determine organic causation

C. Articulation therapy to increase intelligibility

D. Ear training to become aware of the problem

(B) A basic treatment principle is that physical structures be referred for repair prior to initiation of speech treatment, so (B) is the correct answer. (A), (C), and (D) will produce limited clinical results in the absence of an unrepaired cleft so these are incorrect.

Here the examinee was required to make a clinical judgment by applying a known treatment principle for prioritizing events in clinical management. Apply your knowledge of treatment principles to the next question.

The parents of a 4-year-old boy have expressed concern about his dysfluent speech. The speech-language pathologist concludes that the child is exhibiting normal dysfluency. Which of the following most accurately supports this conclusion?

A. The child is too young to have developed dysfluent speech

B. The child displays no associated behaviors

C. The child's speech is 20% dysfluent

D. The child's speech is characterized primarily by whole word repetitions

(D) Whole word repetitions are the major marker of normal dysfluency. Thus, the correct answer is (D). (A) is not a correct statement, and (B) cannot be known from the information given in the question. Dysfluency is a typical marker of early stuttering, so (C) is incorrect.

Analysis Questions

Analytical ability relates to the capacity to think logically in a rule-constrained manner and to use common sense. A typical question may present a set of conditions describing a fictional situation requiring logic and systematic reasoning.

The Praxis may contain questions that require analysis in several different forms. Bloom (1957) gives three forms of analysis: analysis of elements, analysis of relationships, and analysis of organizational principles. The next question is an example requiring both analysis of elements and analysis of relationships.

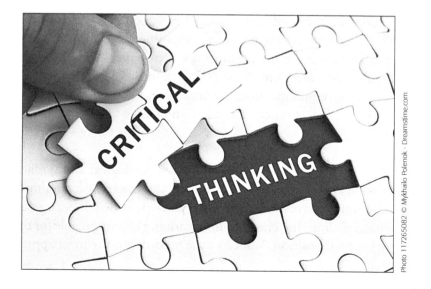

Photo 117265082 © Mykhailo Polenok - Dreamstime.com

Which of the following sentences can be analyzed according to the tree diagram below?

A. An apple keeps the doctor away

B. The tree fell into the water

C. The man went there again yesterday

D. This is the one I like

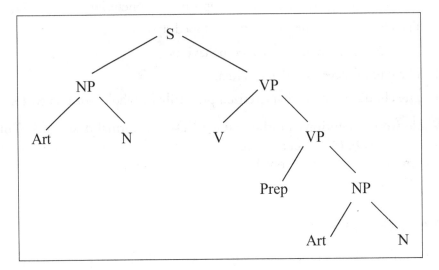

(B) The correct sequence is: **Art** (The) + **N** (tree) + **V** (fell); + **P** (into) + **Art** (the) + **N** (water). Working from the two endpoints of the tree diagram, an article (**Art**) occurs first and a noun occurs last. Hence (C) and (D) are eliminated since the sentences do not end with an article and a noun. Similarly, (A) is eliminated since it does not end with a noun.

Synthesis Questions

Synthesis questions are more difficult than analysis questions because they require the cognitive skill of creativity on the part of the examinee. In addition, the reasoning of the examinee must match the intention of the item writer. Since these questions are presented in multiple-choice format, the examinee must select the single choice that is appropriate for all the requirements of the question. Often, knowledge of specific facts and recall are not needed as much as general knowledge and creativity. Consider the following example:

A 3-year-old boy is diagnosed as having a severe phonological and syntactic disorder. His comprehension ability is within normal limits; however, he has a limited phonetic inventory and multiple errors including final consonant deletion, unstressed syllable deletion, stopping, gliding, and cluster simplification. He is stimulable for the phonemes [p], [t], and [n] in final position. Which of the following is the most appropriate treatment sequence?

I.   Expand phonetic inventory by establishing fricatives [s] and [f]

II. Expand utterance length and use of grammatical morphemes

III. Expand production of initial consonants

IV. Expand inventory of multisyllabic words

A. III, I, II, then IV

B. IV, I, III, then II

C. I, III, II, then IV

D. III, I, IV, then II

(D) From the information presented, the child has both speech and language impairments. The phonological impairments affecting intelligibility (initial consonants) are in need of the most immediate attention, so the first goal is III. Treatment should proceed to the next level of phonological development, fricatives (I) to multisyllabic words (IV) then to utterance length (II). Thus, the correct answer is (D). Use synthesis to answer the next question.

On a test of articulation, a 7-year-old child produces the following utterances:

[f ɑʊ l ɚ] for "flower"

[æ m ə n ə l] for "animal"

Treatment should focus on development of which of the following phonological processes?

A. Labialization

B. Fronting

C. Gliding

D. Metathesis

(D) The examples exhibit that medial consonants that are reversed (/l/ and /w/ in flower; and /m/ and /n/ in animal), which are clear examples of metathesis, so (D) is correct. (A), (B), and (C) are not the phonological processes reflected in the example, so they are incorrect.

Multiple Cognitive Abilities Questions

Some Praxis questions require the use of multiple cognitive abilities. As the number and type of cognitive abilities required for a question increase in complexity, so does the level of difficulty. In fact, many Praxis questions are perceived as difficult not because they tap obscure or difficult subject matter, but because they require sophisticated reasoning or understanding. Contrast the level of difficulty of the next two questions.

I. A hypothetical study of children with articulation disorders is being conducted to determine which of two treatment programs is more effective in remediating a particular pattern of articulatory substitution. Thirty children meeting a number of criteria for inclusion in the study have been selected. The inclusion criteria ensure that the sample is reasonably homogeneous with respect to a large number of variables that might influence the outcome of treatment, such as severity, age, and prior treatment. Which of the following is the best approach to assigning the children to a treatment condition?[1]

A. Randomly assigning half of the children to each condition

B. Allowing the children to select the treatment they prefer

C. Assigning males to one treatment condition and females to the other

D. Giving each child a trial session using each approach and then assigning them to the approach to which he or she responded most favorably

(A) Random assignment to treatment and control groups is conventional in an experimental design. Options (B), (C), and (D) are unacceptable and do not meet the requirements for random assignment.

II. *"No differences exist in the maximal phonatory duration of the vowel /a/ between participants with ataxic dysarthria and matched participants with no history of neurologic disease."*

The statement above is an example of:[2]

A. Independent variable

B. Dependent variable

C. Null hypothesis

D. Research hypothesis

(C) The null hypothesis is a statement of expectancy of no differences between comparison groups. Options (A), (B), and (D) do not meet the definition of a null hypothesis, and are thus incorrect.

The cognitive abilities needed to correctly answer the first question were knowledge plus comprehension, analysis, and synthesis. The second question requires knowledge plus comprehension. For more practice, identify the cognitive abilities needed, and then answer the next question.

Research with language-disordered children has demonstrated that their proficiency with grammatical morphemes is typically below that which would be predicted on the basis of utterance length. This suggests that:[3]

A. Language-disordered children acquire language in patterns of development that are different from those seen in normal children

B. Mean length of utterance is a better index of phrase structure complexity than of morphological knowledge

C. Language-disordered children learn grammatical morphology more slowly than do normal children

D. Grammatical morphology is a relatively unimportant aspect of linguistic competence

(A) This question requires the two cognitive abilities of comprehension and synthesis. The question states that language-disordered children produce fewer grammatical morphemes per unit of utterance length. This is inconsistent with the pattern of normally developing children, who produce more grammatical morphemes within the same utterance length. Thus, the pattern of language development for language-disordered children is different from normally developing children so (A) is correct. (B) and (D) are incorrect statements. (C) is not a logical conclusion of the research finding.

Frequently Asked Questions

■ How can I strengthen my higher-level cognitive abilities for the Praxis?

You use higher-level cognitive abilities in many of your daily activities. The purpose of this chapter is to familiarize you with the specific abilities necessary for Praxis questions. The fact that you are required to use cognitive abilities for the Praxis is what makes the questions appear difficult. The best way to improve these skills is to take practice examinations.

■ What is the best way to put parts together or formulate a novel idea (synthesis) in a short period of time?

You do not need to learn synthesis as a new skill. It is a human cognitive process done naturally and instantaneously. For example, when you answer questions that require the selection of the best treatment strategy, you use synthesis. You must select the correct answer by drawing upon your natural ability to synthesize the information in the question.

■ What strategy is needed to answer synthesis questions?

You do not need to worry about a strategy to answer synthesis questions. Synthesis is one of the cognitive skills that make Praxis questions particularly difficult. If you know the answer, you do not need a strategy. A strategy is a mechanism to help you make a decision when you must guess.

■ How does one analyze a case study without spending too much time on the question?

Analysis is a cognitive process done naturally as you read and comprehend the question. Give analysis questions all the time needed so that you fully understand the question and the answer choices. Timing and reading speed will be addressed in future chapters.

■ You suggested that memorization is not always best, and that one should focus on underlying processes such as application. How should I go about studying for questions like language development?

If you have taken the course, you know the basics. For the Praxis, imagine how language development is applicable in a clinical setting. This is using the cognitive ability of application.

- When approaching questions that require multiple cognitive abilities, is there a particular order to handle the various abilities?

Because multiple are skills needed, these questions appear difficult. You need not be conscious of the cognitive abilities while you take the Praxis. Your intelligent brain does the process for you. For some questions, you may need to analyze before you can comprehend, and then synthesize as a plausible course of action. But this is a natural process.

- I have difficulty with comprehension questions (understanding exactly what the question is asking). Is there a technique that will help me clarify what is being asked?

You are probably familiar with examinations composed of recall questions in which you recognize the answer, or the response is automatic. It is good for you to know your weakness and focus your preparation on taking practice examinations with Praxis-type questions to strengthen your comprehension ability.

- What is the most frequent type of question on the Praxis? Are these questions typically grouped together?

The Praxis is not organized according to cognitive abilities. Rather, it is constructed to reflect the course content areas. The cognitive abilities are embedded in most of the questions to examine critical thinking skills. You will find a variety of cognitive abilities; however, it is not necessary to focus on them during the examination. Instead, use the knowledge of these skills to help you prepare for the Praxis.

- Should one knock out the easier questions first such as knowledge and comprehension, and then go back to the harder ones like analysis and synthesis? Or is it better to recognize the type of question and attack it there?

You might recognize a question as requiring a particular skill. However, it is not recommended that you attempt to skip complex questions. It is best to answer each question in turn and make a guess on difficult questions. With practice, you will perfect your ability to answer difficult questions.

- For analysis questions, how does one know if they are overanalyzing or not analyzing enough?

Analysis is a natural skill. It is possible to overthink a question, that is, read more into the question than what's actually there. Examinees tend to overanalyze when they search for a trick. Praxis questions are not trick questions. As you take practice examinations, be aware of your thought process. If you tend to overanalyze, I recommend practice to change the habit.

- I understand that practice is the best way to correctly answer each type of question, but are there any supplemental materials or exercises to help identify the type of question?

Actually, you do not need to be concerned with the type of question while engaged in taking the Praxis. You will automatically and subconsciously recognize the difficulty level and apply the necessary skill.

- It appears that the Praxis is not a test of clinical knowledge as much as how well one can select the correct answer. Do you feel that this is an accurate test of clinical skill?

It is a bit of both. On one hand it is a test of knowledge. But it is also a test of critical thinking skills that are necessary for clinical practice. This is the reason why Praxis questions differ from classroom exams that test specific knowledge, and why practice with the type of questions is more important than memorizing information.

References

Bloom, B. (1957). *Taxonomy of education objectives: Cognitive domain.* New York, NY: David McKay.

Sources

1. Educational Testing Service. (1982). *NTE programs Ticketron descriptive pool for the Core Battery and Specialty Area Tests* (p. 131). Princeton, NJ: Author.
2. Ibid, p. 131.
3. Johnston, J. (1982). The language disordered child. In J. L. Northern (Ed.), *Review manual for speech, language, and hearing* (p. 287). Philadelphia, PA: W. B. Saunders.

Chapter 4

Reasoning Skills

Standardized tests such as the Praxis require the use of different operations than those that are usually sufficient for classroom exams. In the classroom, instructors write exams to ensure students have acquired the knowledge. Most classroom exams are composed of verbatim recall questions such as the example below:

Prominent shoulder movement is indicative of:[1]

  A. Apnea
  B. Abdominal breathing
  C. Clavicular breathing
  D. Pulmonary distress

(C) is the correct answer since the clavicle corresponds to shoulder movement. Abdominal breathing is normal, and there is no prominent shoulder movement, so (B) is incorrect. Apnea and pulmonary distress are abnormal breathing conditions, but they do not result in prominent shoulder movement, so (A) and (D) are also incorrect.

A common type of question found on the Praxis requires more than sheer knowledge and memory. These questions may resemble verbatim recall questions, but actually much more than knowledge is needed to arrive at the correct answer. Consider the difference between the previous question and the following.

A clinician administers a test of articulation to a 5-year-old child. Upon presentation of the picture of a gun the child refuses to respond, saying, "I can't say that. That's a bad word." To elicit the target sounds, the clinician could most reasonably:

  A. Tell the child that it is not a bad word
  B. Skip the word containing the sound
  C. Insist that it is all right for the child to say the word
  D. Substitute another word containing the sound

(D) is the correct answer since telling the child it is not a bad word (A); skipping the item (B); or insisting that it is all right (C) could pose unanticipated problems in the assessment process.

The above question calls for reasoning skills. The question is somewhat abstract in nature, and perhaps even theoretical. Indeed, more than one of the answer choices might appear to be plausible. Therefore, the examinee must use reasoning skills to select the best answer, or the answer that is most clinically sound.

Reasoning skills are mental operations performed on the answer choices to assist in selecting the intended answer. This chapter discusses various kinds of questions that require reasoning, including 12 reasoning skills listed below. This chapter also discusses a typical question known as the *negative stem question*. It is not necessary to memorize these reasoning skills. The intent of this chapter is to bring them to consciousness so you can use them automatically during the Praxis.

- Classification
- Fusion
- Comparison
- Cluing
- Predicting the examiner
- Focusing
- Abstract reasoning
- Recognizing key words
- Critiquing
- Creativity
- Grouping
- Values

Classification Questions

Questions that require classification are usually theoretical and abstract. The question itself may contain little or no information, while the answer choices contain the necessary facts. Classification questions require three distinct reasoning processes, including:

- discriminating fine differences among answer choices;
- distinguishing quality and quantity aspects among answer choices; and
- prioritizing and placing the answer choices in hierarchical order.

Classification questions often contain words such as *best, least, primary, preferred, major* or *main*. The following is a sample of a classification question. Use the processes above to help you to select the answer.

The practice of speech-language pathology requires informed clinical judgments. Knowing what speech and language disorders can be changed and whether individual clients can change is important for a clinician to:[2]

    A. Implement appropriate clinical services

    B. Determine the best treatment schedule

    C. Know what referrals to make

    D. Offer precise prognostic statements

(A) When the answers are classified in hierarchical order all of the activities reflect appropriate clinical services. Therefore, the correct answer is (A). Taken individually, choices (B), (C), and (D) are incorrect since each is true and there is only one best answer.

    In many classification questions, several of the answer choices may be plausible. However, there is a single best answer. The question may require the examinee to select the option that takes highest priority by classifying the answer choices in hierarchical order, or selecting the answer that is not consistent with the others.

    Note that in some classification questions, the question stem is theoretical or abstract. The appropriate answer choice will also be theoretical and abstract. The wrong answers may be more concrete. Not all classification questions will present a theoretical and abstract choice. However, the examinee must utilize one of the three processes of classification to arrive at the intended answer. With the knowledge you now possess about classification, answer the following question.

In establishing management objectives for a 62-year-old woman who recently sustained a cerebral vascular accident, which of the following should receive the highest priority?[3]

    A. The site of lesion

    B. The rehabilitation framework

    C. The presence of a right hemiplegia

    D. Emotional lability of the client

(B) The rehabilitation framework relates to a complex of circumstances of the clinical situation including those that are biological (A) and (C), as well as those that are psychological (D). To arrive at the correct choice the examinee must classify the answers in hierarchical order. Thus, the single best choice and the correct answer is reflected in choice (B).

Fusion Questions

Fusion questions are the inverse of classification questions. Fusion questions require the examinee to find commonalities among the answer choices and select the one that encompasses the others. Consistent with classification questions, fusion questions can also be theoretical and abstract, and the question may contain little information while much information is contained in the answer choices. However, fusion questions may not necessarily contain qualifiers or superlatives such as *most* or *best*. The following is an example.

To implement speech and language therapy the competent clinician must:[4]

    A. Avoid using a method not previously utilized

    B. Develop rapport with the client

    C. Determine within the first session whether the client will respond to the method

    D. Demonstrate a high level of technical and interpersonal skills

The answer is (D). Answer choices (A) and (C) can be easily eliminated since it is unreasonable to avoid using a method used before and to determine response to intervention in the first session. To arrive at the correct answer, it must be recognized that (D) encompasses the remaining choice (B) and reason that because of developing rapport with the client and having a complete understanding of the disorder, a clinician would demonstrate both technical and interpersonal skills. Use the reasoning skill of fusion to answer the next question.

A clinician conducts procedures to evaluate a school-age child with multiple articulatory errors. When analyzing test results of various measures, the most important observation for classifying the severity of the disorder is:[5]

    A. The number of error sounds

    B. The developmental lag in sound production

    C. Stimulability

    D. Patterns among the errors

The answer is (D). For this question, all of the answer choices appear to be important. So, the correct answer will be the one that encompasses the others. Patterns among the errors (D) encompasses (A) the number of errors, (B) the developmental lag, and (C) stimulability.

Comparison Questions

Similar to classification and fusion questions, comparison questions require specific reasoning operations performed directly on the answer choices. In many cases, the question appears to be a verbatim recall question. However, selection of the correct answer requires more than mere recognition of the answer. Comparison questions require the ability to discriminate differences and evaluate quality, degree, impact, or relevance. Of course, as the name signifies, these questions involve making comparisons among the answer choices as they relate to the information presented in the question. The next question is an example of a comparison question.

Which of the following is most likely to result in hyponasal speech in an individual presenting a cleft palate and previously diagnosed velopharyngeal insufficiency?[6]

    A. Secondary management that occludes the velopharyngeal port

    B. A pharyngeal flap that is excessively narrow

    C. Removal of adenoid tissue

    D. Development of a Passavant's pad

The answer is (D). After reasoning that hyponasal speech results from decreased nasal emission due to <u>increased</u> tissue mass, (B) a narrow pharyngeal flap and (C) removal of adenoid tissue should be eliminated because these conditions result in <u>decreased</u> tissue mass. The examinee must make a comparison between (A) secondary management and (D) Passavant's pad for the greater impact upon hyponasality. The choice presenting the greater effect is (D). Using similar reasoning, answer the following comparison question.

Which of the following is NOT a difference between single case and group experimental designs?

    A. Sample size

    B. Need for control

    C. Length of time needed to observe the dependent variable

    D. Ease of implementation in a clinical setting

The answer is (B). Working through the process of elimination, sample size (A), length of time (C), clinical setting, and (D) are aspects of single case investigations. Since control is necessary for all experimental research the correct choice is (B).

Cluing Questions

Cluing, or recognizing clues within the question, is a reasoning skill that is necessary not only for the Praxis, but also for all exams. Often there are clues within a question that lead to the appropriate answer. Cluing involves the following abilities:

- extracting relevant information from the question;
- recognizing key words or phrases; and
- recognizing the appropriate answer among the choices.

    Cluing is a skill that is particularly important for educated guessing, as well as for changing to the correct answer when you recheck the exam. Clues may be intentional or unintentional. Examinees can develop a skill for recognizing clues within questions. This skill is developed through attention to detail and a conscious effort to find a clue within the question. The following question contains a clue that is perhaps obvious.

Examination of a 6-year-old boy reveals deficits in cognition in addition to articulatory skills. The most useful information for planning articulation remediation is gained from the client's:[7]

A. Physical status

B. Developmental skills

C. Environment

D. Articulatory behavior

The answer is (D). The choices of physical status (A) and environment (C) are unreasonable since they do not relate to articulation treatment. Faulty reasoning might lead an examinee to select developmental skills (B) because it relates to the client's cognition. However, general developmental skills do not contribute to planning for articulation remediation. Therefore, (D) is the correct answer.

The clue in this question is the word *articulatory*, which occurs in both the question and the correct answer. A hasty examinee might overlook this clue.

The following question contains a clue that is not so obvious. First identify the clue, and then answer the question.

Culturally sensitive and relevant procedures of children's language assessment:

A. Have been shown to have no impact on performance of culturally diverse clients

B. Demonstrate that performance of culturally diverse clients is consistent with norms

C. Are virtually impossible to develop and administer

D. Amplify the consistently poor performance of culturally diverse clients

The answer is (B). The examinee should immediately focus on *culturally sensitive* and *relevant* as positive terminology. There is only one positive statement among the choices. Culturally diverse clients show no differences when relevant assessment materials are administered, so the correct answer is (B). The presence of the negative words *no* in choice (A), *impossible* in choice (C), and *poor* in choice (D) make these choices inconsistent with the question; thus, they are incorrect.

Predicting the Examiner Questions

Predicting the examiner is a practice with which students are quite familiar. In the classroom, students learn to recognize the instructor's style and what the instructor emphasizes or thinks is important. Either consciously or subconsciously, students learn to expect what will be presented on an exam.

One important distinction between the Praxis and classroom exams is that the examinee is unfamiliar with the writers of the test questions. One should not assume that the emphasis or camp of thought presented in his or her training institution applies universally, or that the same textbooks for courses are used throughout the nation.

Predicting the examiner involves:

- selecting the universal or most socially acceptable response, and
- using common sense.

Predicting the examiner is an important skill for practicing professionals and those who have been away from academic study for a prolonged time period. Often professionals develop their own personal slant, approach or belief. It is necessary to recognize these and lay them aside for the Praxis. The following is an example of a question that requires the skill of predicting the examiner.

At present, no single theory explains the cause of stuttering because:[8]

    A. There has been no real attention paid to causation theory in recent years

    B. Well-controlled clinical studies have taken precedence over basic research

    C. The population of people who stutter is heterogeneous with considerable variability

    D. Stuttering is not sufficiently prevalent to be adequately studied

The answer is (C). If you selected (A) or (B), you did not predict the examiner because these choices are not consistent with research and these statements would not be found in a professional textbook. You should immediately recognize choice (D) as most incorrect since it is not an accurate statement. Thus, your answer and the correct choice is (C) since the population of people who stutter is heterogeneous.

Use the reasoning skill of predicting the examiner to answer the following question.

Children with language disabilities frequently exhibit concomitant emotional and social disturbances. Which of the following is a true statement concerning clinical intervention for these children?[9]

    A. Since these problems can be expected to resolve with improvement in language skills, they need not be the focus of attention

    B. Since these problems may influence the amount and quality of linguistic input, they should be considered a legitimate focus of language intervention

    C. The clinician must work around these problems since speech-language pathologists are not qualified to address them

    D. Since these problems may disrupt language learning, intervention should not begin until the child achieves emotional health

The answer is (B). It may be your individual opinion or experience that social and emotional problems need not be a focus of attention (A); or should not be considered (C); or that treatment should be delayed (D). However, opinion and experience should not guide your selection. Rather, predicting the examiner requires the textbook or professional response, which is that social and emotional problems are legitimate issues (B).

Focusing Questions

A common type of question found on the Praxis involves focusing, which requires the examinee's keen awareness of what the question is really asking, or what the information in the question implies. Focusing questions may seem complicated at first glance. They may be wordy, narrative clinical descriptions. Focusing questions may also present an example or a case scenario from which examinees must extrapolate particular information or draw specific implications. Thus, they are similar to questions that require the cognitive ability of comprehension. However, another component of focusing is the ability to summarize wordy questions into more concise statements. Consider the difference between the next two questions.

Version I

"No differences exist in the maximal phonatory duration of the vowel /a/ between subjects with ataxic dysarthria and matched subjects with no history of neurologic disease." This statement is an example of:[10]

    A. An independent variable

    B. A dependent variable

    C. A null hypothesis

    D. A research hypothesis

Version II

"No differences exist between the experimental group and control group." This statement is an example of:

    A. An independent variable

    B. A dependent variable

    C. A null hypothesis

    D. A research hypothesis

A statement that no differences exist is known as the *null hypothesis*, so (C) is correct. Independent variable (A), dependent variable (B), and research hypothesis (D) are incorrect because they do not characterize the statement provided in the question.

Perhaps as a result of test anxiety, some examinees may fail to translate version I into its simpler counterpart, version II. Note that the question is not really concerned with ataxic dysarthria or phonatory duration of the vowel /a/. It is a research question, dealing with identifying a null hypothesis.

Use focusing in both the question and the answer choices to answer the following question. HINT: While taking the Praxis it is helpful to make brief notes on your scratch paper and write down important words and phrases.

A 46-year-old female client is self-referred for a vocal examination. She reports that 6 weeks ago she suddenly began to notice a change in her vocal quality and that while speaking she feels she is choking or strangling. Examination with a laryngeal mirror by her family physician revealed no abnormalities. However, the client says that the condition is becoming progressively worse. On the basis of these symptoms, the speech-language pathologist should suspect which of the following conditions?

    A. Laryngeal carcinoma

    B. Contact ulcers

    C. Polyps

    D. Spasmodic dysphonia

If you grasped the concept of focusing, your translation should resemble the following.

A choking, strangling voice is symptomatic of:

    A. Carcinoma

    B. Ulcers

    C. Polyps

    D. Spasmodic dysphonia

The answer is (D). Choices including carcinoma (A), ulcer (B), and polyps (C) are incorrect because they do not result in the symptoms. In spasmodic dysphonia, involuntary spasms in vocal fold vibration produce a choking, strangled voice that is made more severe by stress, so (D) is correct. Use a focusing to answer the next question.

A 76-year-old man has been diagnosed with Parkinson's disease. His head displays a resting tremor that disappears during voluntary movement. He shows considerable difficulty initiating, continuing, and terminating movements required for speech, and his sentences are marked by short bursts of rapid speech. His speaking is also characterized by monopitch, monoloudness, and reduced intensity. Which of the following most accurately characterizes the client's condition?

    A. Hypokinetic dysarthria

    B. Flaccid dysarthria

    C. Ataxic dysarthria

    D. Spastic dysarthria

First, it is important to note that the client presents with Parkinson's disease, which is associated with one type of dysarthria. The question should be mentally reworded as:

Parkinson's disease is associated with which type of dysarthria?

 A. Hypokinetic

 B. Flaccid

 C. Ataxic

 D. Spastic

(A) is the correct answer choice since hypokinetic dysarthria is the only choice associated with Parkinson's disease. (B) is incorrect because flaccid dysarthria is associated with damage to the cranial nerves, (C) is incorrect because ataxic dysarthria is associated with damage to the cerebellum, and (D) is incorrect because spastic dysarthria is associated with damage to the pyramidal tract.

Abstract Reasoning Questions

A common type of question found on the Praxis requires the use of abstract reasoning. These questions usually present information or evidence that the examinee must interpret and draw an appropriate conclusion. In speech-language pathology, abstract reasoning may require clinical judgment; knowledge of and application of diagnostic or treatment principles; and reading and interpreting charts, graphs, spectrograms, tympanograms and audiograms.

Abstract reasoning requires the following abilities:

 ■ discerning the implications of statements or conditions;

 ■ making generalizations to novel conditions;

 ■ applying existing formulas or rules to novel situations;

 ■ understanding relationships among variables presented pictorially; and

 ■ deriving meaning from graphic displays.

The following is an example of a question requiring abstract reasoning.

What would be the most likely effect on resonance of an elongated adenoid pad?[11]

 A. Cul-de-sac

 B. Hypernasality

 C. Hyponasality

 D. Alternating hyponasality and hypernasality

The answer is (C). When there is enlargement of the adenoid pad there is increased tissue mass resulting in reduced nasal emission. The resonance effect of increased tissue mass is hyponasality. (A) is incorrect because cul-de-sac results from a nasopharyngeal blockage, (B) is incorrect because hypernasality results from insufficiency of velopharyngeal tissue, and (D) is an unlikely condition.

For this question the examiner must discern the implication of an enlarged adenoid pad through use of abstract reasoning and logic. The logic must be in perfect one-to-one correspondence with the information in the question and free from overgeneralization and conjecture. Use abstract reasoning for the following question.

Which of the following classes of speech sounds is especially vulnerable to deterioration in the articulation of a postlingually deafened person?[12]

    A. Stop consonants

    B. Front vowels

    C. Final consonants

    D. Diphthongs

The answer is (C). Abstract reasoning is required since the examinee must apply knowledge of the speech characteristics of postlingually deaf persons plus the effects on speech production. Omission of final consonants is a common error in hearing-impaired persons primarily due to reduced force requirements for final consonants and lack of coarticulation effects. Thus, the correct choice is (C). Stop consonants (A), front vowels (B), and diphthongs (D) are not as affected because of the ease of their production.

Key Word Questions

A typical type of question often found on the Praxis involves key words. Key words are defined as superlatives, quantity/quality words, adjectives, or adverbs that are either crucial or merely stylistic within the question. The task of the examinee is to discern the type of key word. Particular key words provide clues to selecting the correct answer. However, some key words may produce ambiguity within the question, and confusion or uncertainty within the examinee. A list of key words used on the Praxis is given below.

Key Words

Best	Used in questions that call for value judgments
	Signals that the answer choices can contain two or more plausible choices
	Used when the answer choice has two components
Most	Used with a qualifier (e.g., *most* reasonable, *most* accurate)
	Almost always an important clue to the answer
	Not essential when used with *probably* and *likely*
Primary	Quantity/quality; signifies the first in a sequence

Major	Always important for selecting the correct answer
Least	Signals the use of classification as a reasoning skill
Preferred	
Main	
Either	Signals the use of classification or fusion reasoning skills
Not	
Might Be	
Primarily	Not key to selecting the correct answer
Typically	Use tends to be stylistic
Commonly	Used with hypothetical cases rather than direct fact questions
Generally	Can be left out grammatically
Usually	Does not provide clues to correct answer
Probably	
Could Be	
Should	

Note that superlatives such as *most* and *best* and quantity/quality words including *major, least, preferred,* and *main* are essential to understanding the question. In addition, words such as *either, not,* and *might be* provide a clue to the appropriate answer choice. Other key words such as *generally* and *primarily* can be confusing to the examinee if too much emphasis is placed on their function within the question. Consider the following questions which contain key words.

Functional articulation disorders are typically caused by:[12]

    A. Poor discrimination ability

    B. Motor incoordination

    C. Unknown factors

    D. Phonological processing problems

The answer is (C). Functional articulation disorders are so designated because they have no apparent organic or nonorganic basis, thus poor discrimination ability (A), motor incoordination (B), and phonological processing (D) are incorrect. The correct answer is (C), unknown factors.

Usually, insertion of the word *typically* in a statement implies that more than one element can be applicable, and the examinee must select the most prominent or most frequently occurring element. Indeed, *typically* literally means *usually*. However, in this question, *typically* is merely stylistic. Consider the next example of a key word that is also stylistic.

Listeners differentiate between various vowel sounds primarily on the basis of:

A. Fundamental frequency

B. Intensity

C. Formant frequencies

D. Duration

The answer is (C). *Primarily* literally means first in a series. In many questions, *primarily* is important because it signifies a classification question. However, this question is not a classification question because the answer choices are either *true* or *false* and cannot be classified sequentially or in hierarchical format. The acoustic patterns that most distinguish vowel sounds are formant frequencies (C). Fundamental frequency (A), intensity (B), and duration (D) are incorrect because they could be identical for each vowel sound.

Critiquing Questions

While it may be said that all questions involve critiquing the answer choices to use the process of elimination, this reasoning ability deserves special mention. Each answer choice is critiqued in relation to the question before selecting the most appropriate answer. The finer elements of critiquing involve the following processes:

- determining the relevance of statements;
- determining and evaluating negative attributes; and
- identifying the worst answer.

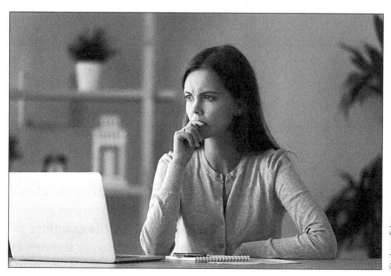

iStock.com/fizkes

Critiquing questions may require a relative amount of general knowledge to answer the question, as reflected in the following question.

Research has identified a sequential pattern of sensorimotor, cognitive, and semantic prerequisites for development of social interactions. In language instruction of severely disabled children, when a client acquires a prerequisite, the clinician could most reasonably:[13]

A. Assume it is available for subsequent activities

B. Assume it generalizes to other response categories

C. Use it to obtain attention for other purposes

D. Use it as a prompt for subsequent responses

The correct choice is (D) since using a learned response as a prompt is clinically defensible. Assumptions that a learned behavior is available for subsequent activities, that it generalizes to other categories, and that it can be integrated with other responses as in (A) and (B) are untenable. Using the response to gain attention (C) is plausible; however, (D) is indisputable since the response can definitely be used as a prompt.

This question requires the examinee to use general knowledge about treatment procedures. In effect, selection of the answer becomes a process of comparison and elimination. The question may be treated as a true/false question, with the intended choice being the single true statement. Yet what makes the above a critiquing process is that the examinee must evaluate each answer choice for its truth or falsity, as well as its relevance. Use critiquing to answer the next question.

Which of the following is the most accurate statement concerning the initial examination of an adult individual who stutters?[14]

A. The examination should be long enough and thorough enough to establish a differential diagnosis and plan of action

B. The examination should involve measures necessary to determine a statement of severity

C. The examination should continue until a procedure with which the client can achieve fluency has been identified

D. The examination should involve a thorough interview with the client's family

(A) The question requires a general knowledge about stuttering assessment. By accurately critiquing each of the choices, the examinee can arrive at the correct answer. Two of the answer choices, unlimited time until a procedure is identified (C) and interview with family (D) are not consistent with basic theory or practice so they can be marked as false. Without using the true/false strategy, the examinee might consider (B) a plausible response since a goal of assessment is to classify severity. However, only one answer is allowed. Since establishing a differential diagnosis and plan of action (A) was initially marked as true, it is the single true statement among the answer choices.

Creativity Questions

Praxis questions frequently present material differently from the way it was introduced in the classroom. Many questions on the Praxis present a clinical scenario in which the examinee's knowledge must be transformed into a plan of action. These questions call for creativity, which is similar to the cognitive ability of synthesis. Creativity involves:

- generating novel thoughts or innovative ideas;

- generating a realistic situation from a theoretical notion; and

- deriving means by which hypotheses can be tested.

For the Praxis, creativity may be necessary for questions requiring location of the site of lesion from specific symptoms, or inversely, ascribing symptoms given the site of lesion. In addition, creativity questions may require the examinee to make a diagnosis or recommendation for treatment. Consider the following question that requires creativity.

A speech-language pathologist examines a 6-year-old boy who was referred for therapy following reconstruction surgery for a cleft palate. The evaluation reveals presence of nasal emission only on /s/ and /z/, with all other pressure consonants produced orally. Which of the following is the most appropriate diagnosis?[15]

    A. Occult submucous cleft palate

    B. Stress velopharyngeal inadequacy

    C. Phoneme-specific velopharyngeal inadequacy

    D. Postoperative velopharyngeal inadequacy

The answer is (C). In the process critiquing the examinee should reason that postoperative structural abnormalities would affect other oral sounds, not specifically /s/ and /z/, therefore submucous cleft (A), stress velopharyngeal inadequacy (B), and postoperative velopharyngeal inadequacy (D), are incorrect. Hence phoneme-specific velopharyngeal inadequacy (C) is the most appropriate selection. Use creativity to answer the following question.

A clinician is most likely to obtain a naturalistic language sample in which of the following communicative settings?[16]

    A. Observing the child while reading in class

    B. Observing the child in dialogue with other children

    C. Observing the child in direct interview

    D. Observing the child's response to standardized language tests

The answer is (B). Of course, this question requires clinical skill in the form of creativity. The examinee must mentally critique each plan of action presented in the answer choices. Observing the child in dialogue with other children (B) is the correct answer since reading (A), indirect interview (C), and testing (D) will not yield naturalistic data.

Grouping Questions

Grouping is a reasoning skill that has been proven as an effective test-taking strategy. Grouping is the inverse of the process of elimination. Answer choices are ruled *in* rather than ruled *out*. Thus, grouping involves finding commonalities among the choices that satisfy the specifications of the question.

Grouping questions are often presented in Roman numeral format. However, grouping questions may also be presented in a format using key words such as *except, not,* and *only*. The correct choice for a grouping question is a combination of items (e.g., I and IV only), or a single item choice that stands out from the other choices (e.g., A. apples, B. oranges, C. grapefruit, D. cabbage). In general, grouping questions are verbatim recall questions. The following are types of grouping questions that are typical for the Praxis.

The elements necessary for sound to be created are:[17]

    I. energy source

    II. compression

    III. transmitting medium

    IV. vibrator

    A. I, II, and IV

    B. I, III, and IV

    C. I and III only

    D. II and III only

The answer is (B). To answer the question, the examinee must recognize that the three necessary elements for sound to be created are energy source (I), transmitting medium (III), and vibrator (IV). Thus, the correct answer is (B) because it the only choice that contains the three elements. A quick and efficient method of selecting (B) is to locate any answer choice that contains the incorrect element, compression (II). As a result (A) and (D) would be immediately eliminated because they contain choice II. (C) is incorrect because it does not contain a required element, vibrator (IV). The following is an example of a different grouping question.

All of the following are parts of a neuron EXCEPT:[18]

    A. Axon

    B. Soma

C. Ganglion

D. Dendrite

The answer is (C). The examinee must either rule out the single false choice or rule in each choice individually. A proven strategy for attacking this type of question is to treat each choice as a true or false statement. The answer is the single false choice, or (C). Axon (A), soma (B), and dendrite (D) are the components of the neuron so these are incorrect.

Values Questions

In speech-language pathology, examinees are frequently required to make clinical judgments on the basis of values reflected in the questions or the answer choices. Typical values reflected in the Praxis are:

- law abidance;
- fairness and equity;
- protection of client rights;
- professional decorum;
- team spirit;
- cooperation with other professionals;
- objectivity; and
- respect for the scientific method.

It is extremely important to read the American Speech-Language-Hearing Association (ASHA) Code of Ethics and the Speech-Language Pathology Scope of Practice. These documents can be located on the ASHA website. This knowledge will be required for questions in administration. These questions are very easy, but the knowledge is so specific that it is usually impossible to answer the questions without having read the documents. The following is a sample question that reflects the values of the profession.

In dysphagia intervention, the primary concern of the speech-language pathologist is:[19]

A. The client's comfort

B. The client's respiratory status

C. The family's wishes

D. The client's nutritional status

The answer is (D). Given the values of the profession, the examinee should immediately recognize (D) as the correct answer since the highest value of the profession is the life and quality of life of the client. Hence, the client's comfort (A), respiratory status (B), and family's wishes (C) are important, but not primary considerations.

Answer the next question using your sense of professional values.

Which of the following is the most accurate statement regarding intervention procedures for language disabilities?[20]

A. Language-disordered children should be given precedence in the caseload over language-delayed children.

B. Therapeutic intervention is useless in cases that have a neurologic basis.

C. The initial focus of therapy should be the development of language structures rather than social or cognitive skills.

D. Early intervention for all children is essential.

The answer is (D). This question reflects a basic societal belief, as well as the law. Thus, the correct answer is (D) since it is both lawful and reflects the professional value for clinical practice. Giving precedence to language disorders (A), and focusing on language structures (C), are unreasonable actions. (B), intervention as useless in neurologic cases, is incorrect because this statement is inaccurate.

Negative Stem Questions

Negative stem questions often contain the words *not, least,* or *except*. These questions are sometimes difficult for examinees because they require a sudden cognitive shift. While there may be few, if any, negative stem questions on the Praxis, knowledge of the strategies for attacking these questions is helpful. The best strategies for negative stem questions are:

- Write the negative word on your scratch paper to reemphasize its significance
- Select the answer choice that is incompatible with the others
- For **NOT** questions, use the true/false strategy, marking each answer on your scratch paper as either *(T) true* or *(F) false*. Then group the choices selecting the single true choice or the single false choice. With the answer choices marked, the single true or false answer is immediately visible as in the following example.

Which of the following is **NOT** a characteristic associated with apraxia of speech?[21]

A. Client awareness of errors **T**

B. Client frustration **T**

C. Left hemiplegia **F**

D. Right facial weakness **T**

(C) is the correct answer because apraxia of speech is associated with right hemiplegia; therefore, the statement is false. Other characteristics include right facial weakness (D); and the client shows awareness (A) and frustration (B). Thus, these statements are true. Using a similar reasoning process and the true/false strategy, answer the next question. But first, translate the question as a positive statement, then mark each answer *(T)* or *(F)*.

Which of the following is **NOT** related to vocal resonance?[22]

A.	Tongue height	T	F
B.	Oropharyngeal constriction	T	F
C.	Velar elevation	T	F
D.	Vocal fold elasticity	T	F

The answer is (D). Whether you marked the answer choices as *true* or *false* or used a process of elimination, your answer should be (D) since vocal fold elasticity is a property of the larynx and is not associated with resonance. Tongue height (A), oropharyngeal constriction (B), and velar elevation (C) are aspects of the vocal cavity and thus are indeed associated with resonance.

Final Note

The discussion in this chapter is not intended to provide an overall strategy or approach for the Praxis. It is important to remember that you do not need to memorize the types of questions presented in this chapter. It is important, however, to perform the various reasoning operations when needed to assist in selecting the correct answer choice **only** when you are uncertain and must make a guess. Naturally, if you recognize the correct answer you will not need any strategy to assist.

Frequently Asked Questions

- When using some of the reasoning techniques, I find myself focusing on the technique and running out of time. How can I make a smoother transition to incorporate the techniques?

The chapter does not imply that these are new techniques to be learned. Chances are you already use the operations spontaneously and subconsciously. Let this chapter bring these natural operations to consciousness for use only when you are unsure of the answer. If you know the answer, you will not need any technique, thus utilizing your time optimally.

- Finding commonalities among the choices is a skill I find challenging, especially "All of the Above" questions. Is there a specific strategy to attack this type of question?

Fortunately, the Praxis is unlikely to contain "All of the Above" questions. However, you will encounter Roman numeral questions. It is appropriate to use the true/false strategy as well as classification as a reasoning skill.

- Is there a good strategy for deciphering unfamiliar technical words?

If the unfamiliar word is in the answer choice, it is best not to choose that answer. If the unfamiliar word is in the question and you do not know the material, then guess and go to the next question.

- How important is critiquing? How do you know when to use a particular reasoning skill?

All the processes discussed in the chapter are equally important. They are processes to use only when you are unsure of the answer. If you have practiced, as long as you are aware of the necessity to use the skills, you will use them instinctively according to the demands of the question.

- When answering a question you are not familiar with, should you eliminate answers and then use the reasoning skills, or do you use the reasoning skills to eliminate answers?

Actually, if you are eliminating answers you are using reasoning skills. Both ways are helpful.

- What is the best strategy for values questions—memorization, gut feeling?

Utilize your gut feeling based in knowledge. For example, you need not memorize the ASHA Code of Ethics, but you must be familiar with it. Then apply your knowledge to the question.

- Besides grouping and negative stem questions, does the true/false method work for any of the other types of questions?

Indeed, the true/false strategy can assist in eliminating wrong answers and narrowing the choices in many types of questions.

- Can't cluing get you in trouble by picking an answer that is too obvious?

Don't allow cluing to be your main approach. Cluing is a method of taking an educated guess. Use cluing and the other reasoning skills only when you are unsure of the answer. If you know the answer, you do not need to use cluing.

- Aren't the clinical application answer choices subjective? I know the questions present extreme answer choices, but can't some answers be perceived differently by different people?

Perhaps, but there is always a single best answer, which is usually the same as the textbook response.

- Knowing key words is great, but can I really internalize the words under the pressure of time? Won't that cause me to overanalyze the question?

Hopefully you will have practiced many questions before you take the Praxis. Practice enables you to internalize these reasoning skills so they are automatic when you take the exam.

- When critiquing should I select the answer according to my clinical experience, or choose the answer professionals would deem as correct?

It is not wise to use your clinical experience. Rather, select the textbook answer or the answer professionals would deem as correct.

- When focusing, if an answer choice includes information that was stated indirectly in the question should I choose this answer?

Yes. In choosing this answer you will be using comprehension and focusing, as well as cluing.

- What reasoning skill would be best to use for case study questions?

Unfortunately, it is not possible to align the question format to a specific reasoning skill. When you need to guess, perform the reasoning operation according to the demands of the question.

- I have difficulty with Roman numeral questions. How safe is it to select "All of the Above?"

This is not a safe strategy. It is better to eliminate answer choices based on your knowledge. The true/false strategy can be helpful in narrowing your choices.

- In fusion questions, are there key terms that aid in eliminating answer choices? I'm having difficulty with the examples provided.

For fusion questions, eliminate choices that are insufficient alone to answer the question, as well as any two answers that are both plausible. Select the single answer that represents the commonalities, is most complete, and encompasses the others.

- Would it be wise to completely ignore the key words that are unrelated to selecting the answer?

The point of key words is not to ignore them but to differentiate between those that are important and those that are merely stylistic.

- I have difficulty with classification and fusion questions. How can I develop the skills to discriminate between answer choices?

Read the sections of this chapter again until you fully grasp the concepts. Seek opportunities to practice these skills.

- In answering a reasoning question, would thinking of a response before reading the answer, then picking the response that closely resembles your answer, prove more effective than reading the choices and then deciding?

That will work in most cases, especially when you know the answer. But be careful not to use your clinical experience to select the answer instead of selecting the textbook response.

- I think cluing works great sometimes. Are there questions that present similar words in the answer choices just to throw you off?

The Praxis does not intentionally insert trick questions. However, not all questions that appear to hold a clue can be answered by cluing. If you know the answer, there is no need to use cluing. Cluing, as all the reasoning skills in this chapter, is useful to help you select the intended answer when you are uncertain.

Sources

1. Nation, J., & Aram, D. (1982). The diagnostic process. In J. L. Northern (Ed.), *Review manual for speech, language and hearing* (p. 138). Philadelphia, PA: W. B. Saunders.
2. Ibid. p. 138.
3. Ibid. p. 139.
4. Ibid. p. 139.
5. Bankson, N., & Bernthal, J. (1982). Articulation assessment. In J. L. Northern (Ed.), *Review manual for speech, language and hearing* (p. 204). Philadelphia, PA: W. B. Saunders.
6. Educational Testing Service. (1982). *NTE programs Ticketron descriptive pool for the Core Battery and Specialty Area Tests* (p. 132). Princeton, NJ: Author.
7. Educational Testing Service. (1995). *A guide to the NTE Speech-Language Pathology Specialty Area Test* (p. 132). Princeton, NJ: Author.
8. Guyette, T., & Baumgartner, S. (1989). Stuttering in the adult. In J. L. Northern (Ed.), *Study guide for handbook of speech-language pathology and audiology* (p. 168). Philadelphia, PA: B. C. Decker.
9. Johnston, J. (1982). The language disordered child. In J. L. Northern (Ed.), *Review manual for speech, language and hearing* (p. 286). Philadelphia, PA: W. B. Saunders.
10. Op. cit. Educational Testing Service. (1982). p. 131.
11. Peterson-Falzone, S. (1989). Speech disorders related to craniofacial structural defects: Part 2. In J. L. Northern (Ed.), *Study guide for handbook of speech-language pathology and audiology* (p. 120). Philadelphia, PA: B. C. Decker.
12. McReynolds, L., & Elbert, M. (1982). Articulation disorders of unknown etiology and their remediation. In J. L. Northern (Ed.), *Review manual for speech, language and hearing* (p. 212). Philadelphia, PA: W. B. Saunders.
13. Turton, L. (1982). Communication and language instruction for severely handicapped children and youth. In J. L. Northern (Ed.), *Review manual for speech, language and hearing*, (p. 241). Philadelphia, PA: W. B. Saunders.
14. Op. cit. Guyette, T., & Baumgartner, S. (1989). p. 168.
15. Op. cit. Peterson-Falzone, S. (1989). p. 130.
16. Payne, K. (1989). Speech and language difference and disorders in multicultural populations. In J. L. Northern (Ed.), *Study guide for handbook of speech-language pathology and audiology* (p. 269). Philadelphia, PA: B. C. Decker.
17. Freeman, F. (1982). Stuttering. In J. L. Northern (Ed.), *Review manual for speech, language and hearing* (p. 25). Philadelphia, PA: W. B. Saunders.
18. Larson, C., & Pfingst, B. (1982). Neuroanatomic bases of hearing and speech. In J. L. Northern (Ed.), *Review manual for speech, language and hearing* (p. 10). Philadelphia, PA: W. B. Saunders.
19. Robbins, J. (1989). Dysphagia and disorders of speech. In J. L. Northern (Ed.), *Review manual for speech, language and hearing* (p. 306). Philadelphia, PA: W. B. Saunders.
20. Waryas, C., & Crowe, T. (1982). Language delay. In J. L. Northern (Ed.), *Review manual for speech, language and hearing* (p. 281). Philadelphia, PA: W. B. Saunders.
21. Kearns, K., & Simmons, N. (1989). Motor speech disorders: The dysarthrias and apraxias of speech. In J. L. Northern (Ed.), *Study guide for handbook of speech-language pathology and audiology* (p. 152). Philadelphia, PA: B. C. Decker.
22. Op. cit. Educational Testing Service. (1995). p. 122.

Chapter 5

Reading Comprehension

This chapter is particularly important for individuals for whom English is a second language and reading proficiency in English is not high. This chapter is also useful for individuals who do not perform well on timed, structured exams.

Difficulty of exam questions depends, in part, on the reading level of the question. Reading level is associated with the elaborateness of language, syntactical complexity, and amount of technical jargon in the questions and answer choices. Reading comprehension is a distinct process from the cognitive abilities and reasoning skills needed for successful test performance. Reading comprehension requires several complex mental processes that must be in simultaneous operation during reading. The following is a diagnostic checklist of the mental processes for reading comprehension.

- Concentration
- Absorption of meaning
- Knowledge of technical jargon
- Reflection
- Contemplation
- Evaluation (agreement/disagreement)
- Recall
- Association/identification
- Appreciation for metaphor, symbolism, style, sarcasm

Each of these mental processes is under the reader's direct control. But to improve reading comprehension, the examinee must be aware of the extent to which these processes are or are not in operation, and practice those processes that are found to be diminished or lacking. Only through practice can the mental processes be developed and enhanced to improve reading comprehension during the Praxis.

The next two questions can be used to test your reading comprehension. Read each question and note your use of the mental processes in the checklist presented previously.

Question I.

Below are two excerpts of opinions on the same issue by two eminent scholars in communication disorders.

A. *The position statement suggests that the eradication of the dialectal utterance is inappropriate. Further, it suggests that the speech-language pathologist may also provide elective clinical services to nonstandard English speakers who do not present a disorder. According to the position statement, the role of the speech-language pathologist for these individuals is to provide the desired competence in standard English without jeopardizing the integrity of the individual's first dialect. I believe we do a significant disservice to social dialect speakers if we employ this approach—the do-nothing strategy. Surely it is time for us to assume a more positive and vigorous stance than advocated in the position paper* (Adler, 1985).

B. *According to the position statement, standard English is the language of specific institutions within society. Further, it is stated that individuals who seek assistance in learning standard English should have the option of receiving such services from a speech-language pathologist. Imposing standard English as a second dialect presumes that nonstandard English speakers cannot learn to code-switch without mandatory clinical intervention. What Adler proposes is not far removed from days past when dialect speakers were routinely enrolled in speech therapy to have their dialects "corrected"* (Cole, 1985).

The two views of the scholars are best characterized by which of the following statements?

    A. They disagree over whether speech pathologists should provide clinical intervention to dialect speakers

    B. They disagree over whether dialect speakers should receive mandatory clinical intervention

    C. They disagree over whether standard English should be the language taught to dialect speakers

    D. They disagree over whether dialect speakers can learn standard English

The answer is (B). Since it is clear that the scholars disagree, in selecting the answer the examinee can first eliminate (D) since it is untenable. The remaining choices require the examinee to comprehend the source of the disagreement. There is one best answer that specifies that the source of the disagreement is whether clinical services for dialect speakers should be mandatory.

Question II.

Below are two excerpts of opinions on the same issue by two eminent scholars.

A. *The question focuses on psychosocial, cognitive and linguistic development. We all have a responsibility to provide children with unrestricted access to all the tools available for optimal growth and lifelong success. Learning sign does not relegate a child to the deaf world, as commonly thought. Conversely, learning speech does not automatically admit a child to the hearing world. Many deaf signers have fully developed speech capabilities and function successfully in both the deaf and hearing worlds, which are by no means distinct and independent of each other. Children with implants who have parallel visual language development opportunities have greater ability to interact with deaf peers and adult role models. This, in turn, leads to a healthier sense of identity and psychosocial development, for success in both communities. Without such opportunities, implanted children could well wonder where and with whom they feel most at ease when they reach adulthood (Bloch, 2000).*

B. *A child who receives a cochlear implant does not have normal hearing, just as a child who is hard of hearing and uses hearing aids does not have normal hearing. Both children are, in fact, functionally hard of hearing. There is no evidence that children who are brought up to be part of Deaf culture are somehow psychologically better off than deaf children who are brought up in the larger world. Access to spoken language offered by cochlear implants provides individuals with the ability to function with greater independence and maximize their life opportunities. Ultimately, this is a choice that parents make for their children. Parents in America and elsewhere still have the final say in how they wish to have their children brought up. Whether parents decide to have their child brought up as part of Deaf culture or as part of the larger world is a decision that parents should make with full knowledge of the decision-making and its consequences (Sorkin, 2000).*

The two views of the scholars are best characterized by which of the following statements?

    A. They disagree over whether using cochlear implants affects psychological well-being

    B. They agree that using cochlear implants improves psychological well-being

    C. They disagree over whether cochlear implants should be imposed on deaf children

    D. They disagree over whether children with cochlear implants can learn sign language

The answer is (B). Since it is clear that the writers agree on some issues and disagree on others, it is important to search for the points of overlap. The examinee can utilize the true/false strategy to arrive at the correct answer, (B). (A) is incorrect since both agree that cochlear implants impact psychological well-being. (C) and (D) can be eliminated since they are not true statements.

If you did not select (B) as your answer to both questions, pay particular attention to the discussion in this chapter and return to the questions after you have completed the chapter to test your grasp of reading comprehension.

Reading is a form of communication in which the reader is the receiver of a written message. In reading comprehension, it is the task of the reader to decipher the message as it was intended. Since the author of the written message is not present during the communication to add nonverbal cues and clarify misunderstandings, it is expected that the conventions of writing have been adhered to so that the reader's comprehension of the message is facilitated. If the writer and reader have the same expectations for the written message, the message is more likely to be received as intended. Hence, reading comprehension can be facilitated if the reader has some knowledge of the conventions of writing.

On the Praxis, short passages or clinical scenarios are presented for the examinee to interpret. It is important for the examinee to know that paragraphs are usually developed around one central theme. Usually a topic sentence, which is the first sentence, introduces the main theme of the paragraph. However, depending upon the writer's style and purpose for communication, the topic sentence may be implied, or may even be stated at the end of the paragraph.

In paragraphs where the topic sentence is stated first, there are usually several successive sentences that bear a relationship to the topic sentence. These sentences provide supporting detail and further development of the main idea. The final sentence may either be a culminating statement or a connecting statement for the next paragraph.

Paragraphs that have a topic sentence stated last are usually organized in such a manner as to build to a climax. Generally, the first sentence is the most minor in the sequence in which more and more information is presented.

There are two principles of organizational patterns for paragraphs: coordination and subordination. In coordinate paragraphs, all supporting sentences carry the same weight. In paragraphs organized by subordination, each successive sentence adds information or support to the previous sentence. Paragraphs may also be organized as a mixture of coordinate and subordinate styles.

For passages that contain more than one paragraph, the organization usually follows a pattern of progression from the general to the specific. Paragraphs may be arranged to produce an additive effect, in which more information on the topic is presented in each successive paragraph. With this knowledge, when the reader is able to discern the general organization of the communication, reading comprehension is enhanced.

Emphasis

An important distinction between reading and listening is the nonverbal cues available to the receiver of the message. Listening, of course, requires fewer mental processes than reading because vocal and visual cues may accompany the spoken message.

Not all questions will provide clues as to the author's emphasis. The reader must practice reading for emphasis until it becomes a natural process. An effective method for practicing reading with emphasis is to read each passage aloud, emphasizing the words as in delivering a speech. Read aloud the preceding question, placing vocal emphasis where necessary. Then practice reading comprehension using the following question.

How is one to study an organ such as the brain? The major approach, of course, is to study its components and then try to learn how they function together. This is done primarily in animals rather than in humans. The principles of neuronal function are remarkably similar in animals as far apart as the snail and the human; most of what is known about the nerve impulse was learned in the squid. Even the major structures of the brain are so similar in, say, cats and humans that for most problems it seems to make little difference which brain one studies. Moreover, neurobiology is notable for the wide range of approaches and techniques that have been brought to bear on it, from physics and biochemistry to psychology and psychiatry. In no other branch of research is a broad approach so essential, and in recent years it has begun to be achieved.[1]

The following statements are related to the information presented above. Based on the information given, select:

(A) If the statement is supported by the information given

(B) If the statement is contradicted by the information given

(C) If the statement is neither supported nor contradicted by the information given

A B C   1. Much can be understood about the human brain from animal studies

A B C   2. The theory of cerebral localization is unfounded

A B C   3. A snail's brain contains all the major structures found in the human brain

A B C   4. The science of neurobiology has an interdisciplinary basis

A B C   5. In terms of neuronal function, the human brain is more complex than other species'

1. (A)   2. (C)   3. (C)   4. (A)   5. (B)

If you answered any of the above questions incorrectly, read the passage using the diagnostic checklist to analyze your problems. Continued practice may be indicated to improve your reading comprehension.

Reading Speed

Not much can be done to improve your basic reading speed at this stage of your life. Throughout your many years of practice with reading, you have probably reached a plateau where your speed is now optimal for comprehension of what you read. To the contrary, your reading speed can be diminished if: (1) the material is above your reading level, (2) your concentration is lax, (3) the topic is boring, or (4) complex material is introduced for the first time. Reading speed can also be reduced if you are mentally fatigued, frustrated, or anxious.

The importance of getting rest before the exam cannot be overstated. With proper rest, if your mind becomes sluggish during the exam, you will have the power to perk up. However, if you have not had sufficient rest, you will become progressively more sluggish. With proper rest, you can also increase your reading speed for short periods of time, or for short passages, and maintain your level of comprehension.

Timing is an important aspect of the Praxis. It is not recommended that you speed read the Praxis to finish, but you can speed read short questions where selection of the answer requires only recognition. Therefore, you can save time to use toward reducing your speed for the more wordy, complex, and difficult questions. The following recommendations will aid in improving your reading efficiency on the Praxis.

- Be mindful of the time limitation, but do not speed read the exam. Vary your reading speed for different questions.

- Glance at each question first to decide whether the question can be read more quickly, or if you should reduce your reading speed.

- Increase your speed for short questions and for material that is familiar to you.

- Read at your usual speed for wordy, complex questions, or questions that require more concentration.

Using the tips above answer the next question and note the number of seconds from the beginning until you make your answer selection.

Record Start Time _____

Stacy is 3 years old. Her parents are concerned that her speech and language performance is not on par with that of her older siblings during their 3rd year. In the speech and language evaluation, it was observed that Stacy pulled her mother, or pointed or placed her mother's hand on objects she desired. There was limited verbal communication; however, Stacy displayed echolalia in response to questions and commands. She would stack four blocks, but showed no response to dolls, cars, and attempts at book reading, with a preference for repetitive, self-stimulating behaviors. From the above information, the speech-language pathologist should most appropriately:

A. Plan a treatment regimen to address language delay

B. Refer to a psychologist to confirm autism spectrum disorder

C. Defer treatment for 6 months, then conduct further observation

D. Administer additional standardized tests of speech and language

Record End Time _____   **Total Seconds** _____

The answer is (B). The main key to the suspicion that the client should be referred for assessment of autism is in the repetitive and self-stimulating behaviors. (A) is incorrect because although some behaviors seem to suggest language delay, the symptoms of autism are paramount. (C) is incorrect because the client's behaviors warrant immediate attention. (D) is incorrect because further testing is not likely to yield usable results since the child exhibits limited attention and verbal responses.

The maximum time to answer this question should be 48 seconds. If you exceeded the maximum time, review this chapter extensively and seek additional practice to improve your reading speed.

Chunking

You were probably taught to read by a method that stressed reading every word individually. Perhaps initially you were taught to recognize particular letter and syllable combinations to synthesize a whole word. As you became a more skillful reader, you were able to eliminate this strategy and recognize whole words by sight, and thus improve your reading skill and speed immensely. This strategy is known as *chunking*.

Chunking can be utilized to increase your reading speed for the Praxis. However, the chunking strategy is used for word combinations rather than syllable and letter combinations. You can learn a strategy to recognize particular word patterns and combinations on the Praxis that eliminates the need to read each word individually. The following are syntactical and word combinations that are typical for the Praxis. Become familiar with these phrases to increase your reading speed.

Which of the following

Which of the following is the least

Which of the following is the most

Which of the following is the most appropriate

Which of the following is the most likely

Of the following, which

. . . the most appropriate

. . . the most effective

. . . the most likely

Most accurately

A speech-language pathologist

The speech-language pathologist should

The speech-language pathologist should most appropriately

A clinician

The next step

What is the primary

What is the first

What is the next

The primary purpose

. . . is generally

. . . is primarily

. . . is typically

. . . is the most important

. . . is the best

. . . is an example of

. . . is known as

The primary reason

It can be reasonably concluded that

The initial

It is also important to become familiar with the structure and format of typical Praxis questions. Each Praxis question is presented in traditional multiple-choice question format, or as an incomplete statement. This organization has two implications for reading speed. In many cases, an examinee can learn to anticipate what must be done to arrive at the correct answer. For example, for traditional question format, the examinee can learn to mentally formulate a tentative answer. Holding this answer in mind, the mental process becomes one of matching the printed answer choice to the examinee's tentative answer. When the correct answer is recognized, the examinee need not spend excessive time evaluating the answer choices.

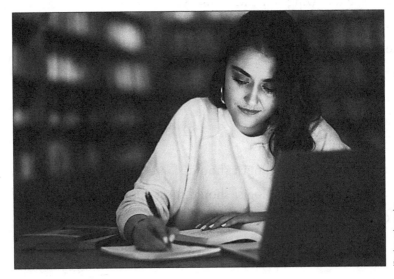

For questions of the same length that are presented as incomplete statements, the examinee must spend additional time evaluating each answer choice for its appropriateness. Thus, comparatively, incomplete sentences may require more time than questions in the traditional question format. The format can also be helpful for distinguishing questions that can be read quickly from those that will require greater time and concentration.

Preview Strategy for Increasing Reading Speed

A useful strategy in some cases is to glance at each question before you conduct a thorough reading. If the answer choices are presented as one word or short phrases, the examinee can glance at the answer choices to obtain a preview or sense of the topic of the question. Psychologically, this preview strategy may also have the effect of providing cues to questions presented as incomplete statements and rapid recognition for matching the examinee's tentative answer for questions presented in typical question format. However, it is **not** recommended that you take the time to read the complete answers for every question, because this will only cost you valuable time in the long run. Remember, you should preview each question, but **only** read the answer choices that are composed of one word and short phrases. Using the following question, practice the preview strategy by first glancing at the short phrase answer choices below, presented without the question.

A. Group intervention

B. Articulation drills

C. Visual action therapy

D. Melodic intonation therapy

Now read the question presented below and return to the answer choices to select the answer.

Which of the following is the most appropriate treatment for a client with aphasia who has extremely poor comprehension, repetition, and verbal production?[2]

A. Group intervention

B. Articulation drills

C. Visual action therapy

D. Melodic intonation therapy

The answer is (C) Visual action therapy emphasizes visual strengths in clients with poor comprehension, so (C) is the correct answer. (A) is incorrect because group intervention is inappropriate for clients with poor comprehension. Articulation drilling (B) will not address comprehension problems, so (B) is incorrect. (D) is incorrect because melodic intonation therapy focuses on increasing fluency.

Reading Comprehension Practice Exercise

Follow the steps indicated and select the answer to the next question.

Step 1: Read the question, chunking the bolded phrases.

Assessment of a preschool-age child has suggested that the child is at risk for stuttering. Numerous part-word repetitions and some hesitations are presented, but the child seems unaware of the dysfluencies. However, the parents are very concerned and put a great deal of pressure on the child to "stop stuttering." The home environment is very structured, and the parents talk quickly and interrupt each other. In this situation, **the speech-language pathologist** can **most appropriately** suggest **which of the following** kinds of treatment?[3]

Step 2: Mentally formulate a tentative answer.

[*Don't call attention to the problem*]; [*Delay treatment*]; [*Provide parental counseling*].

Step 3: Compare your tentative answer to the choices.

   A. Direct intervention focused on reducing the child's rate of speaking
   B. Direct intervention focused on increasing length and complexity of utterances
   C. Parent counseling, environmental manipulation, and monitoring of fluency
   D. Psychological counseling for all family members by physician referral

Step 4: Eliminate choices that are inconsistent with your tentative answer.

   A. Direct intervention for rate
   B. Direct intervention for length and complexity
   D. Psychological counseling for all family

Step 5: Match your tentative answer to the correct answer.

The answer is (C). Since the child is at risk for stuttering, it is best not to make the child aware of it because awareness increases anxiety and, therefore, may increase it, so (C) is correct. The parents' anxiety can be communicated to the child, so the parents should be counseled. The child should be monitored to determine if direct intervention will eventually be necessary. (A), (B), and (D) are incorrect because direct intervention and psychological counseling are not always necessary with preschool children. Practice using the sequential steps in the next question.

Head trauma resulting from motor vehicle accidents, falls, sports injuries, or physical insult often leads to changes in a child's cognitive functioning that can affect behavior and learning problems. Which of the following is the most appropriate strategy for the speech-language pathologist to begin to work with a child who has suffered head trauma?[4]

   A. Begin with large-group activities to facilitate appropriate interaction skills and progress to one-on-one treatment.

   B. Rekindle the child's premorbid concept of being normal before progressing to more challenging tasks.

   C. Begin with rote language tasks with high levels of success before progressing to more challenging tasks.

   D. Begin with elicitation of complex linguistic structures and regress to simpler linguistic material only if the child is unable to perform complex tasks.

The answer is (C). Performing familiar rote language tasks associated with high levels will help the child cope with post-trauma cognitive disorganization and will establish a positive basis for intervention involving more challenging activities; thus, the correct answer is (C). The large-group activities described in (A) may be too overstimulating and should not necessarily precede one-on-one intervention, so (A) is incorrect. (B) is also incorrect because it describes intervention that may or may not be appropriate, but it is not typically within the practice domain of the speech-language pathologist. (D) is incorrect because the approach described is inappropriate since it would undermine the child's confidence.

Frequently Asked Questions

■ It is stated that speed reading could be utilized for short questions but not throughout the exam. Should one start off with speed reading short questions and come back to the lengthy questions?

Such a strategy is not necessary. It is more prudent to answer each question in succession.

■ When practicing chunking and speed reading, should we begin with timing ourselves?

If you know that you are a slow reader, it would be wise to practice to increase your speed for easy and short questions. Long and complex questions require greater concentration and should be read at your usual speed.

■ If speed reading decreases comprehension for specific content, is it okay to read at normal reading rate?

Absolutely. Accuracy is more important than finishing the exam.

- I would think chunking might lead to misreading the question due to anticipating, and not thoroughly reading the question. Am I being overly paranoid?

Chunking does not entail skipping the words or phrases, but rather not reading each word individually. Chunking should only be done with the familiar phrases in this chapter.

- I am having difficulty setting a steady reading pace. I become anxious about time and fail to pay attention to the details. I know that through practice I can increase speed and accuracy. Are there any other suggestions?

You are probably experiencing test anxiety. A future chapter will provide suggestions for coping with test anxiety.

References

Adler, S. (1985). Comment on social dialects. *ASHA, 27*(4), 46.

Bloch, N. (2000). Cochlear implants. *Sound and Fury.* Retrieved from http://www.pbs.org/wnet/soundandfury/cochlear/debate5.html

Cole, L. (1985). Comment on social dialects. *ASHA, 27*(4), 47.

Sorkin, D. (2000). Cochlear implants. *Sound and Fury.* Retrieved from http://www.pbs.org/wnet/soundandfury/cochlear/debate5.html

Sources

1. Hubel, D. (1974). *The brain* (p. 4). New York, NY: W. H. Freeman.
2. Tye-Murray, N. (2010). Auditory habilitation and rehabilitation. In D. Ruscello (Ed.), *Review questions for the speech-language pathology Praxis examination* (p. 228). Maryland Heights, MO: Mosby-Elsevier.
3. Educational Testing Service. (1995). *Guide to NTE Speech-Language Pathology Specialty Area Test* (p. 92). Princeton, NJ: Author.
4. Op. Cit. Educational Testing Service. (1995). p. 110.

Chapter 6

Mental Preparation

Effective test-taking requires a combination of cognitive, affective, and behavioral strategies. This section will discuss the affective qualities related to mental and psychological preparation for successful performance on the Praxis.

Throughout your educational experience, you have probably been admonished to get plenty of sleep on the night before an exam. This advice is appropriate for the Praxis. The reason is simple. Since you will be taking the Praxis for more than 2 hours, it is likely that within this time you will become both mentally and physically fatigued. If you have had the proper amount of rest, you can rely on your energy reserve to refresh yourself. If you have not had the proper rest, it is likely that you will have no energy reserve. Thus, you may become even more fatigued. This, of course, can have a deleterious effect on your performance. Test anxiety is a major contributor to mental fatigue. The proper amount of sleep will also help you combat test anxiety.

Believe it or not, diet is also an important component of mental and psychological preparation. Be certain to eat a healthy breakfast on the morning of the exam. But do not introduce new foods that your body is not accustomed to processing. If you do not typically drink coffee, don't drink it on the day of the exam. Similarly, if you drink coffee daily, continue to do so because your body is conditioned to receive it. But don't overextend either your food or coffee intake. Follow your daily routine as closely as possible with regard to wake-up time and the amount, timing, and types of foods and beverages. That second cup of coffee "just to calm your nerves," combined with a high level of anxiety, may prove deleterious to your performance.

Vitamins, minerals, and herbs that improve concentration and mental alertness are recommended for intake beginning at least 30 days before the exam. This will allow your body to adjust and produce effects spontaneously. Taking new vitamins and pills, especially caffeine, on the day of the exam is not recommended. Nor should caffeine pills be consumed to help improve your study. Of course, you should not consume alcohol or stimulants on the day before the exam.

Similarly, don't introduce new foods to your diet on the days prior to the exam. Be aware of how particular foods react with your body chemistry and avoid foods that may cause allergic reactions or bloating, constipation, or discomfort. Do not alter your usual eating routines. If you must be on a weight loss diet, either begin well before the exam or after the exam. Naturally, you should not overeat before the exam.

Maintain your normal exercise routine. Tense or sore muscles can cause discomfort and distract from your concentration. Practice relaxation routines in the days prior to the exam so they become natural and easy. Remember that you will be sitting in one posture and constricting muscles that have not been exercised continuously. Practice deep breathing exercises to relax chest and shoulder muscles and reoxygenate blood cells and brain neurons. Deep breathing can also serve to refocus your thoughts for better concentration. You can relax the muscles of your hand and fingers by flexing and releasing as many times as necessary.

Utilize the power of positive thinking to your benefit. In the same manner that athletes claim the home field advantage and pep rallies boost morale, keep your associations positive and seek the cheerful support and encouragement of others. Pump yourself up for the challenge. Banish negative thoughts, fear, dread, doubt, and anxiety. Devise your personal affirmations and believe in them wholeheartedly. If you are religious, know the power of prayer. Also seek the powerful prayers of others. Create a positive vision of the exam situation and environment. Finally, claim the victory by planning your own celebration activity and look forward to it.

Test Anxiety

Test anxiety is that unsettling, unpleasant, discomforting feeling one may experience in anticipation of, or during, an exam. Research has documented that some anxiety is helpful for test performance. Test performance can actually improve as anxiety increases, but only up to a point. Some individuals respond to test anxiety as a positive force. This phenomenon can result in enhanced performance for all examinees if it is harnessed and controlled. Positive performance depends on knowledge of test-taking strategies, self-confidence, whether previous experiences have been successful, and whether significant others feel confident about your performance.

With extremely high levels of anxiety, performance begins to decline. If there are factors operating to cause you to anticipate failure, test anxiety can become maladaptive and interfere with performance.

Examinees may experience distress, confusion, fear, physical malaise, and worry. As a result, they might respond with ineffective coping strategies and decreased problem-solving ability. High levels of test anxiety occur when: (1) the situation is seen as difficult, challenging or threatening; (2) the individual is uncertain of his or her ability to handle the task at hand; and (3) the individual expects or anticipates failure.

Because of the discomfort, individuals who experience high test anxiety are often strongly motivated to find means of escape and resort to various coping mechanisms such as withdrawal, projection, and rationalization.

Withdrawal can take many forms. For example, even though students are encouraged to take the Praxis near the end of their graduate study, many do not comply. Also, if students take the Praxis near the end of their graduate study and do not succeed, instead of taking the exam at the next opportunity, quite frequently they wait many months, if not years, to retake the exam. By then, their command of knowledge is much less than it would have been closer to the end of their graduate study.

Another frequently used defense mechanism is projection. Some repeat examinees are convinced that their past failure was deliberately planned by the "powers that be" who developed the test and set the passing score. As a result, they tend to believe the misconceptions about the Praxis, which in turn, perpetuates test anxiety.

Test your level of test anxiety with the following exercise.

Praxis Anxiety Prediction Scale

1. During an exam, I tend to forget some of the information I know:
   A. Often
   B. Sometimes
   C. Rarely
   D. Never

2. After an exam, I can recall some answers that I could not remember during the test:
   A. Often
   B. Sometimes
   C. Rarely
   D. Never

3. During an exam, I worry about whether I have enough time to finish:
   A. Often
   B. Sometimes
   C. Rarely
   D. Never

4. During an exam, I can't wait to be done so I can leave and do something pleasurable:
   A. Often
   B. Sometimes
   C. Rarely
   D. Never

5. Before an exam, I can't sleep well:
   A. Often
   B. Sometimes
   C. Rarely
   D. Never

6. Before an exam, I worry about whether I studied enough:
   A. Often
   B. Sometimes
   C. Rarely
   D. Never

7. During an exam, I worry that other people are finding the test to be easier:
   A. Often
   B. Sometimes
   C. Rarely
   D. Never

8. During the test, I find some frustrating questions that are stupid or irrelevant:
   A. Often
   B. Sometimes
   C. Rarely
   D. Never

9. During a multiple-choice test, I find that I know the answer but my answer is not one of the choices:
   A. Often
   B. Sometimes
   C. Rarely
   D. Never

10. During an exam, I get annoyed by other people's behaviors:
    A. Often
    B. Sometimes
    C. Rarely
    D. Never

11. During an exam, I become concerned about whether I'm doing poorly:
    A. Often

B. Sometimes

C. Rarely

D. Never

12. During an exam, I feel as though I need to take a break:

    A. Often

    B. Sometimes

    C. Rarely

    D. Never

13. During an exam, I think about all the other things I would rather be doing:

    A. Often

    B. Sometimes

    C. Rarely

    D. Never

14. During an exam, I tend to daydream:

    A. Often

    B. Sometimes

    C. Rarely

    D. Never

15. During an exam, I worry about what will happen if I fail:

    A. Often

    B. Sometimes

    C. Rarely

    D. Never

16. During an exam, I spend too much time on difficult questions:

    A. Often

    B. Sometimes

    C. Rarely

    D. Never

17. During an exam, I misinterpret the meaning of some questions:

    A. Often

    B. Sometimes

    C. Rarely

    D. Never

18. During an exam, I sometimes feel like I should just give up:
    A. Often
    B. Sometimes
    C. Rarely
    D. Never

19. After the test, I feel that I should have done better:
    A. Often
    B. Sometimes
    C. Rarely
    D. Never

20. After the test, I find that I made too many errors that could have been avoided:
    A. Often
    B. Sometimes
    C. Rarely
    D. Never

Scoring   A = 3   B = 2   C = 1   D = 0   Total _____

Scoring Interpretation

46–60   High test anxiety

31–45   At risk for test anxiety

0–30   Low risk of test anxiety

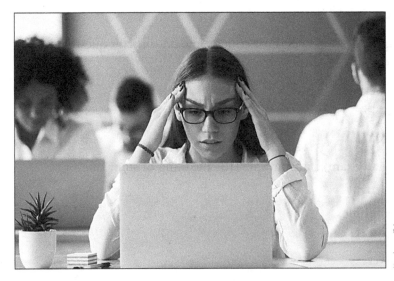

Tips to Combat Test Anxiety

- **Distrust myths you have heard about the test.**

Read all the information about the test. Review the misconceptions and facts in Chapter 2.

- **Don't focus on past failures.**

If you have taken the Praxis previously without passing, realize that the study and preparation undertaken with this book will benefit greatly. Adopt an attitude of confidence.

- **Don't base your experience on the reports of others.**

Each individual's experience is different. Test-taking skills, preparation, and study are as important as grade point average.

- **Begin preparation well before the test date.**

Success with practice questions and exams, plus mental preparation, will boost confidence.

- **Visit the student counseling center.**

Professionals can help you with test anxiety and help you plan coping strategies, budget study time, and adopt relaxation techniques.

- **Don't cram.**

Complete all study one day before the exam. Relax the night before the exam. Get your usual hours of sleep.

- **Meditate before the exam.**

If meditation is not for you, physical exercise is recommended.

- **Do mental warm-up exercises before the exam.**

A warm-up exercise need not be related to the Praxis. The purpose of warm-up is to exercise your brain.

- **Avoid drugs and other stimulants.**

If possible, delay taking medications that might cause drowsiness or take then on the night before the exam. Don't take sleep-inducing medications on the night before.

- **Be sure to feed the parking meter for ample time.**

The Praxis lasts 2.5 hours; however, you may spend more than 3 hours in the exam environment.

- **If possible, visit the test location before the date of the exam.**

This will allow you to find the best travel route and scout for parking.

- **Visualize yourself taking the exam with ease.**

This is known as creative visualization. Manifest the vision during the exam.

- **Avoid toxic people.**

Find a trusted and supportive exam buddy to accompany you to the testing center. Avoid negative and test-anxious people. Select a different testing center if necessary.

- **During the first minute, write down mnemonic devices and other points you have memorized on your scratch paper.**

Test anxiety can cause memory blocks; writing these on the back of the exam booklet will ease anxiety.

- **After setting a pace for the first half-hour, don't focus on time.**

Excessive worry about time can interfere with concentration.

- **Set a comfortable approach to the exam for the first 10 questions.**

Using the strategies in this book will assist.

- **Take a very brief relaxation break.**

When you feel anxious, take a minute to regain composure. This will be beneficial even if you do not finish the exam.

- **Practice thought blocking.**

If your mind wanders, return to the task at hand. If negative thoughts enter, immediately replace them with positive affirmations.

- **Use anxiety to your advantage.**

Remember that a little anxiety is a stimulant and it can be beneficial to performance.

In the days before the exam, use the following exercise to rate your preparation for the Praxis.

Are You Prepared for the Praxis?

1. Have you read the pertinent information about the Praxis?
   A. No
   B. Maybe
   C. Yes

2. Are you comfortable with the date and time of your exam?
   A. No
   B. Maybe
   C. Yes

3. Are you familiar with format, instructions, and areas covered by the exam?
   A. No
   B. Somewhat
   C. Yes

4. Have you reviewed the course content necessary for the areas of the exam?
   A. No
   B. Somewhat
   C. Yes

5. Have you studied material from courses you have not taken?
   A. No
   B. Somewhat
   C. Yes

6. Have you studied the areas of the exam that are most difficult for you?
   A. No
   B. Somewhat
   C. Yes

7. Have you reviewed undergraduate coursework?
   A. No
   B. Somewhat
   C. Yes

8. Do you know the strategies for guessing on the exam?
   A. No
   B. Somewhat
   C. Yes

9. Have you read the ASHA Code of Ethics and Speech-Language Pathology Scope of Practice?
   A. No
   B. Somewhat
   C. Yes

10. Are you confident of your knowledge base?
    A. No
    B. Somewhat
    C. Yes

11. Have you released negative thoughts about the exam?
    A. No
    B. Somewhat
    C. Yes

12. Have you adopted a positive mental outlook?

    A. No

    B. Somewhat

    C. Yes

13. Have you practiced with questions similar to those on the exam?

    A. No

    B. Somewhat

    C. Yes

14. Have you practiced the necessary cognitive requirements for answering the type of questions on the exam?

    A. No

    B. Somewhat

    C. Yes

15. Can you answer most questions in less than 48 seconds?

    A. No

    B. Sometimes

    C. Yes

16. Can you implement effective stress-reduction activities?

    A. No

    B. Somewhat

    C. Yes

17. Can you postpone concern about other worries in your life and focus on the exam?

    A. No

    B. Maybe

    C. Yes

18. Do you possess a high level of motivation to perform as well as possible?

    A. No

    B. Somewhat

    C. Yes

19. Are you prepared to make accurate and appropriate clinical judgments based on textbook knowledge?

    A. No

    B. Not sure

    C. Yes

20. Are you able to apply theories or facts to real-life hypothetical situations?
    A. No
    B. Maybe
    C. Yes

21. Can you factor out pertinent details of a clinical case to draw appropriate conclusions?
    A. No
    B. Somewhat
    C. Yes

22. Can you derive relationships among details and draw clear conclusions?
    A. No
    B. Somewhat
    C. Yes

23. Did you score fairly well on other standardized tests (e.g., SAT, GRE)?
    A. No
    B. Almost
    C. Yes

24. Does your reasoning reflect the attitudes, values, current practices, and professional standards of the profession?
    A. No
    B. Maybe
    C. Yes

25. Can you sublimate your personal beliefs in favor of the consensus of the profession?
    A. No
    B. Somewhat
    C. Yes

26. Have you practiced the reasoning skills involved in answering the type of questions on the exam?
    A. No
    B. Somewhat
    C. Yes

27. Do you fully comprehend material when you read it quickly?
    A. No
    B. Somewhat
    C. Yes

28. Does your academic and clinical background provide an adequate basis for understanding the intricacies of the questions on the exam?
    A. No
    B. Maybe
    C. Yes

29. Can you interpret charts and graphs and make appropriate conclusions?
    A. No
    B. Maybe
    C. Yes

30. Are you familiar with the various research designs?
    A. No
    B. Somewhat
    C. Yes

31. Can you identify dependent and independent variables given a description of a methodology?
    A. No
    B. Maybe
    C. Yes

32. Can you identify independent and dependent variables in a research study?
    A. No
    B. Maybe
    C. Yes

33. Are you familiar with various test-taking and guessing strategies?
    A. No
    B. Somewhat
    C. Yes

34. Have you practiced various test-taking and guessing strategies with success?
    A. No
    B. Somewhat
    C. Yes

35. Are you familiar with the rule for answering a set number of questions per time period?
    A. No
    B. Not sure
    C. Yes

36. Have you achieved a passing score on a practice test?

    A. No

    B. Maybe

    C. Yes

37. Do you recognize the importance of rest and appropriate nutrition on test performance?

    A. No

    B. Maybe

    C. Yes

38. Have you given maximum effort toward preparation for the exam?

    A. No

    B. Somewhat

    C. Yes

Scoring

A = 1

B = 2

C = 3

Score Interpretation

38–56	Ill prepared Review coursework, take the practice exam and practice test-taking skills
57–75	Not prepared Practice test-taking skills. Retake the practice exam.
76–94	Minimally prepared Practice test-taking skills.
95–114	Well prepared Good luck!

Frequently Asked Questions

- Should we study until the morning of the Praxis, or is there a cutoff time to just stop and focus on relieving stress?

If you tend to have test anxiety, it is recommended that you take some time before the test for mental preparation. The need to study until the morning of the exam should be eliminated by beginning your preparation well before the exam date. Even if you have not studied as much as you would like, give yourself a break and gain confidence from the preparation you have conducted.

- If I have a mental block, is it best to guess for the sake of time or try to regain my thoughts to give the best possible answer?

Actually, these choices are one and the same. Guess to save time. Flag the questions you want to revisit after you complete the exam. Your thoughts will be clearer when you no longer worry about finishing.

- Besides taking three deep breaths, is there anything else we can do during the test to relieve stress?

Stress management is an individual process. There are many, many ways to relieve stress. You should find the method that works best for you. Do this well before the exam and practice so it is natural and effective during the Praxis.

- It is recommended that one stops to take a break. Is it okay if I take a minute to regroup? I tend to get distracted when I am sitting for a long period of time.

If you experience test anxiety, it is advisable to take a short break at your seat to relieve stress. This is different from taking an extended break to leave the room. It is okay to take a time out if you are distracted, but immediately return to the task at hand.

- Should I avoid coffee completely, or is it safe to have a cup if I have anxiety?

Don't avoid coffee if you drink it regularly. If you don't normally drink coffee, don't use it as a stimulant or to relieve anxiety.

- I have heard it suggested that we divide tests into small parts. Can this apply to the Praxis?

That may be a personal strategy for you. So, if you need to take a mental break after every 25 questions, for example, this might be useful.

- I've heard that one strategy for relieving anxiety is to bounce around among the questions as opposed to answering them in order. Is this a good idea?

Although this might be a coping strategy for particular individuals, I would not recommend it as a general approach to the exam for everyone. Keeping track of the questions as you bounce around is an unnecessary cognitive demand.

- How do you know when you've studied enough? I never feel like I truly know and retain everything.

You will not need to know everything for the Praxis. When you are performing well on practice tests, you can be confident that you are well prepared.

- When anxiety sets in, is it smart to perform relaxation exercises that may be out of the norm for you?

No. Actually, you should find out what works best for you and practice it before the exam.

- What is the best way to avoid drawing a blank during the exam? Is it better not to study the night before, or the morning of, the exam?

Mental blocks might not be avoidable, but it is possible to return your focus to the exam if you have the appropriate attitude and rest. To avoid drawing a blank, get your normal rest the night before. If you do encounter a blank, take a break or flag that question and return to it later.

- What is the best way to block out negative thoughts that contribute to test anxiety?

You probably cannot prevent yourself from having negative thoughts, but you can control their effect. Determine not to give in to them. Replace negative thoughts with positive affirmations.

- I have done several practice questions finishing within the given amount of time, but that still doesn't make me any less anxious. What do you suggest?

You may not need to be completely free of anxiety. Test anxiety is similar to stage fright. A little anxiety can actually help your performance. As long as the anxiety is not debilitating, it can actually be used to your advantage.

Chapter 7

Test-Taking Strategy

Perhaps in the exercise in Chapter 1 you noted that you perform better with fill-in, true/false, or matching questions rather than multiple-choice questions. It is important to realize that the single point of distinction among all these question types is the format.

Matching and multiple-choice questions both demand that you recognize the correct answer in a pool of different choices. These questions allow you to eliminate some choices. True/false questions are similar in that you must make a single choice but only between two options. Fill-in questions require immediate recall of information.

If you are adept at one type of question, you can use the same skills to improve your performance with multiple-choice questions simply by changing your perception. In your mind, a multiple-choice question can easily become a fill-in, matching, or true/false question.

As you approach each question, first formulate a tentative answer in your mind before you select the answer choice, as you would for a fill-in question. Next, search for your answer among the options, as you would for a matching question. Remember that the answer may not be stated exactly as your formulation, but the idea should be consistent. In many questions, this procedure will not be possible. Therefore, holding your original answer in mind, you can test each option against yours, as you would a true/false question. You should even strike through the options as you eliminate them.

The following is a general approach for improving your performance on the Praxis.

- Move at a quick yet comfortable pace through each question of the exam. Because guessing will increase your score, attempt to answer every question, guessing if you are unsure.

- When you encounter a question you know nothing about, TAKE A RANDOM GUESS. Some individuals prefer to use the same letter for each guess. This strategy is a good as any. The probability of being correct when you guess is 1 out of 4.

- If you think you know the answer, but do not immediately find your answer among the choices, eliminate as many choices as possible. Use the reasoning skills discussed in Chapter 4 to select the best answer. If you can eliminate all but two answers, guess wisely between the two. If you know something about the question and can eliminate some choices, try to eliminate all but two and then guess wisely. Flag the question to return to when you complete the exam. Keep a mental record of the number of questions you flagged for return.

- If you know the material within the question, you should flag it if:
  - ☐ You have a memory block.
  - ☐ The question takes more time than it should.
  - ☐ You do not grasp the meaning.
  - ☐ The question seems to be ambiguous.
  - ☐ The meaning of a chart, graph, or audiogram is not apparent.
  - ☐ You are certain of your answer, but your answer does not appear among the choices, or you disagree with the answer choices.
  - ☐ There seems to be more than one plausible answer.
  - ☐ You wish you had studied this area more.

- If there is time remaining when you complete all the questions, return to the questions you flagged. Don't start at the beginning and attempt to redo the entire exam.

- If there is time still remaining after you return to the questions you flagged, check the questions from the beginning. Be sure to utilize all the time you are given. Do not leave the exam before time is called.

WORD OF CAUTION! From the practice examination in Appendix A, you should have gained a pretty good notion of the kind of test taker you are. For example, if you changed an answer, did you change from the right answer to the wrong answer? If so, don't change your first guess. Only change if you are certain that you are choosing the correct answer.

The questions in the next exercise are recall questions that require specific knowledge. Select the appropriate letter if you know the answer. Answer each question in succession without stopping. If you are unfamiliar with the question content, practice strategies for guessing by marking the [X] or [?] located below each question. Return to questions you marked with a [?] and change the answer only if you are certain that your change is correct.

1. Which of the following may best describe learning disabilities?[1]

   A. A generic term that refers to a heterogeneous group of disorders

   B. A specific language problem with some concomitant dysfunction in reading

   C. A homogeneous group of children with primary problems in reading and writing

   D. A specific problem that is restricted to academic skills acquisition

X ?

2. Which of the following areas of linguistic knowledge seems to present the greatest difficulty for the language-disordered child?[2]

   A. Phrase structure rules

   B. Lexical meaning

   C. Grammatical morphology

   D. Relational semantics

X   ?

3. What type of prosthetic device is often used in cases of inadequate velar movement?[3]

   A. Palatal lift

   B. Palatal plate

   C. Speech bulb

   D. Feeding obturator

X   ?

4. An adult male has had 3 weeks of voice intervention for contact ulcers but remains dysphonic. The vocal behavior most likely responsible for his poor progress is:[4]

   A. A speaking fundamental frequency around 125 Hz

   B. Beginning voice production with a hard glottal attack

   C. Shortened vowel durations in speech

   D. Poor velopharyngeal closure

X   ?

5. Which pathological condition only occurs along the medial border of the posterior of the glottis?[5]

   A. Vocal nodules

   B. Vocal polyps

   C. Contact ulcer

   D. Myasthenia laryngis

X   ?

6. The variable with the greatest predictive power for prognosis in articulation learning is:[6]

   A. Stimulability

   B. Oral and facial motor skills

   C. Speech sound discrimination

   D. Laterality

X   ?

7. Which of the following clinical hypotheses would lead to the most specific clinical design?[7]

    A. John is cognitively impaired

    B. James' language disorder is related to a maturational delay

    C. Bob's semantic disorder interacts with his pragmatic and syntactic problems

    D. Mrs. Smith has Broca's aphasia resulting from a cerebrovascular accident

X ?

8. Disturbances in execution of the motor speech act due to muscular paresis are classified as:[8]

    A. Aphonia

    B. Apraxia

    C. Aphasia

    D. Dysarthria

X ?

9. All of the following appear to be viable explanations of developmental language disorders EXCEPT:[9]

    A. Difficulties with attention control

    B. Symbolic deficits

    C. Neurological dysfunction

    D. Restricted exposure to the physical environment

X ?

10. All of the following are treatment approaches for young children beginning to stutter EXCEPT:[10]

    A. Negative reinforcement

    B. Eliminating physical stress

    C. Creating rewarding communicative situations

    D. Reducing sources of emotional distress

X ?

1. (A) *Learning disabilities* is a general term that refers to a group of disorders characterized by functional difficulties in acquiring academic skills and failure to achieve academic standards inconsistent with the learner's age and intellectual ability. Learning disorders may be apparent in other areas than reading and writing, so (B) and (C) are incorrect. (D) is incorrect because learning disorders are not restricted to adolescents.

2. (C) While language disorders may manifest in each of the areas of phrase structure rules (A), lexical meaning (B), and relational semantics (D), grammatical morphology (C) is the area wherein most specific errors are found. Therefore, the correct answer is (C).

3. (A) To ameliorate inadequate velar movement that results in hypernasal speech, a palatal lift prosthetic device is used to physically provide closure to a weakened velopharyngeal port by displacing the soft palate; therefore the correct answer is (A). A palatal plate (B), speech bulb (C), and feeding obturator (D) are devices used when there is velopharyngeal inadequacy or structural deformities rather than muscle weakness, so these choices are incorrect.

4. (B) A hard glottal attack is the only factor listed that is commonly considered to be etiologically related to contact ulcers, so (B) is the correct answer. Fundamental frequency (A), vowel duration (C), and velopharyngeal closure (D) do not affect contact ulcers; therefore, they are incorrect.

5. (C) Contact ulcers are lesions on the posterior third of the vocal fold. Thus, the correct answer is (C). Anatomic in origin, contact ulcers form when the vocal folds collide against each other at the point of the vocal process of the arytenoid cartilage. Vocal nodules (A) and vocal polyps (B) are incorrect because these lesions may occur in any location of the vocal folds. Myasthenia laryngis (D) is incorrect because it is a muscular disability.

6. (A) Stimulability refers to the ability to produce a target sound when provided with a model. It has the most predictive power for prognosis in articulation learning. Because oral and facial motor skills (B), and perceptual abilities (C) are present and thus will not need to be learned, these answers are incorrect. Laterality (D) is generally unrelated to articulation, so (D) is also incorrect.

7. (D) The answer choices present various etiologies for clinical intervention. (D) is correct because Broca's aphasia implies a specific set of symptoms that can be targeted in treatment and specific treatments are available. Cognitive impairment (A) , language delay (B), and semantic disorder (C) are nonspecific etiologies.

8. (D) The only accurate answer that refers to muscular paresis is dysarthria. Aphonia (A) is loss of voice due to laryngeal nerve damage. (B) and (C) are incorrect because apraxia (B) is a motor speech disorder that affects motor planning, resulting in problems in sequencing sounds and syllables, and aphasia (C) is a global term for several receptive or expressive language disorders related to listening, reading, and writing.

9. (D) The obvious answer is (D), restricted exposure to the environment. Since attention control (A), symbolic deficits (B), and neurological dysfunction (C) are clearly related to developmental language disorders, these answers are incorrect.

10. (A) Negative reinforcement differs from punishment in that negative reinforcement entails cessation of an aversive stimulus. Negative reinforcement is

not a treatment approach in young children. Therefore (A) is the correct answer. Eliminating stress (B), rewarding communicative situations (C), and reducing sources of emotional distress (D) are typical treatment approaches for young children beginning to stutter, so these are incorrect.

Recommended Test-Taking Behaviors

> Read all instructions and follow directions specifically as indicated.

> In your approach to questions, strive to fit into the status quo rather than think of yourself as an exception.

> Adopt an organized and systematic manner of thinking and reasoning.

> Minimize the effects of your personal experiences, beliefs, or values. Think of the common experiences of the profession.

> Actively combat any stress that you feel, particularly if you have negative thoughts. Return your focus to the task at hand.

> Use deductive reasoning in selecting your answers.

> Think hard; concentrate. Be aware of time. Conserve time.

> Place value on precision—only one right answer.

> Read all answer options before making your final choice.

> Even if you have not studied as much as you would have liked, rely on your mental powers and the general knowledge you possess to give you confidence. Never let yourself feel defeated.

> Think of the exam as a means to an end, not as a barrier to your progress.

> Adopt the attitudes, values, and mental outlook of the question writers. Think of yourself not as a student whose ideas are either right or wrong, but as a knowledgeable, integrated professional whose ideas are accepted.

> Pay attention to detail. Expect that every detail counts.

> Apply universal diagnostic and therapy principles. Don't focus on exceptions.

> Look for underlying meanings and implications, but draw conclusions based only on a strict and logical interpretation of the evidence presented.

> Remember specific facts. Let your memory of specific tasks serve as the basis for choosing or eliminating answers in the present context. In other words, use what you know. Recall and relate the small details.

> Assume an active role in the exam, not a passive role. That is, put your mind to work to figure out the answer. Don't expect the answers to come to you.

> Once you have selected an answer, mentally defend your choice using sound reasoning and the facts you know. If your choice is not defensible, choose another option and know that it is correct.

Behaviors NOT Recommended

Do NOT:

- ❖ Reinterpret the directions.
- ❖ Take a casual approach to the exam.
- ❖ Rely on your global, contextual memory from the classroom.
- ❖ Expect the exam to present information the way it was presented in the classroom. Be prepared to apply information in a different context.
- ❖ Change your answers unless you are certain your first choice is not correct.
- ❖ Answer questions based on your personal clinical experiences. The Praxis presents textbook clinical scenarios and requires basic textbook knowledge. Subordinate your personal experiences and utilize generic academic knowledge.
- ❖ Utilize strategies that you have heard about but not practiced, or have not proved to be effective for you.
- ❖ Leave any questions unanswered.

Frequently Asked Questions

- ■ Is it smart to answer the question in my head first and then choose the closest answer, or should I read all the answers?

You won't be able to formulate an answer for every question, so it is wise to read all the answer choices for every question and compare the choices. Even for questions for which you can formulate an answer, you should always read all the answer choices, eliminating the wrong answers and then selecting the best answer.

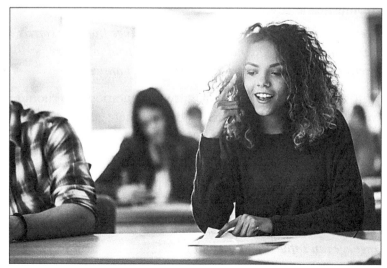

iStock.com/skynesher

- If I run out of time while checking the questions I flagged for review, should I just use the guessing strategies to make sure that I beat the timer?

Check only those questions you flagged to return for review. The computer will record the questions you flagged, as well as the remaining time. Use this information to decide if you can reach all of the questions. If you cannot review all of them in the time remaining, work quickly to review as many as you can.

- My personal guessing strategy is to always mark (C). Is that a good strategy?

You probably won't get many of those questions correct. When you must take a wild guess, you can increase your chances by varying your choices. Do this only for questions you know you do not know. For questions where you have some knowledge, take an educated guess and flag that question for review.

- When unsure, I tend to read a question more than once. Should I continue this, or is it better to mark it and forget about the answer?

If you reread most of the questions, you won't have time to finish. You may need to reread a few questions for clarity. If you're still confused about the question, guess and flag it for review.

- I know you recommend not leaving the exam before time is up. If I should finish before time, do you recommend reviewing all the questions, or should I just sit and relax?

Certainly, if you have completed your review well before time, it is permissible to leave. If you have time to review all the questions, be careful not to use the excess time to change answers unless you are certain that your first answer was wrong.

- Should I be worried if I finish before time is up?

Not necessarily. This may mean that you have used time wisely.

- When should you go back and change the answer, and when should you just go with your first answer?

Many examinees who change answers find that they change from the correct answer to the incorrect answer. Examinees who do not change answers tend to perform well. Don't change unless you are certain that you are changing to the correct answer.

- I know it is suggested that once you answer a question you should not second-guess yourself and change the answer, but are there any exceptions to this rule?

If you are guessing when you change the answer, it is better not to change. Change only when you are certain that your first answer was an error.

- Given the length of time to complete the Praxis, does the average person have enough time to review the whole exam?

The Praxis is designed to be completed in 2.5 hours. Factors such as reading speed, mistakes, and second language can influence your timing.

■ If the Praxis is a computerized exam, how is it possible to go back to answers that we may have skipped?

You will be able to flag questions you want to review.

Sources

1. Guildford, A. (1989). Language disorders in the adolescent. In J. L. Northern (Ed.), *Study guide for handbook of speech-language pathology and audiology* (p. 196). Philadelphia, PA: B. C. Decker.
2. Johnson, J. (1989). Specific language disorders in the child. In J. L. Northern (Ed.), *Study guide for handbook of speech-language pathology and audiology* (p. 285). Philadelphia, PA: B. C. Decker.
3. Peterson-Falzone, S. (1989). Speech disorders related to craniofacial structural defects: Part 2. In J. L. Northern (Ed.), *Study guide for handbook of speech-language pathology and audiology* (p. 130). Philadelphia, PA: B. C. Decker.
4. Larson, D., & Pfingst, B. (1982). Neuroanatomic bases of hearing and speech. In J. L. Northern (Ed.), *Review manual for speech, language and hearing* (p. 12). Philadelphia, PA: W. B. Saunders.
5. Reed, C. (1989). Voice disorders in the adult. In J. L. Northern (Ed.), *Study guide for handbook of speech-language pathology and audiology* (p. 223). Philadelphia, PA: B. C. Decker.
6. McReynolds, L., & Elbert, M. (1982). Articulation disorders of unknown etiology and their remediation. In J. L. Northern (Ed.), *Review manual for speech, language and hearing* (p. 212). Philadelphia, PA: W. B. Saunders.
7. Nation, J. (1982). Management of speech and language disorders. In J. L. Northern (Ed.), *Review manual for speech, language and hearing* (p. 145). Philadelphia, PA: W. B. Saunders.
8. McNeil, M. (1982). The nature of aphasia in adults. In J. L. Northern (Ed.), *Review manual for speech, language and hearing* (p. 263). Philadelphia, PA: W. B. Saunders.
9. Johnson, J. (1989). The language disordered child. In J. L. Northern (Ed.), *Study guide for handbook of speech-language pathology and audiology* (p. 256). Philadelphia, PA: B. C. Decker.
10. Goldstein, R. (1982). Neurophysiology of hearing. In J. L. Northern (Ed.), *Review manual for speech, language and hearing* (p. 65). Philadelphia, PA: W. B. Saunders.

Chapter 8

Time Utilization

For the Praxis, you will have 150 minutes to answer 132 questions. Literally, this means that you have slightly more than 1 minute per question. But actually, if you intend to have enough time to recheck the questions flagged for review, you have less than 1 minute—48 seconds to be exact. Surprisingly, 48 seconds do not pass as quickly as you might think relative to exam taking. Some questions may take as little as 5 or 10 seconds to read and select the answer. Other questions, of course, may take longer than 48 seconds.

Time utilization is directly related to reading speed. Before the Praxis, it would be prudent to determine your reading speed as well as the speed at which you answer exam questions. Without speed reading, use the next question as a diagnostic timing exercise. Give yourself 48 seconds to read the question and mark your response without speed reading.

Timing Exercise

Record Start Time _____

A 5-year-old boy with cerebral palsy exhibits multiple articulation errors characterized by slow and labored speech, general slurring, and some problems with saliva control. The vowels and plosives are generally recognizable. The sibilants and fricatives are inconsistent: sometimes intelligible, sometimes distorted, and sometimes omitted. The boy's parents want their son's speech to improve. The speech-language pathologist can most appropriately utilize which of the following strategies?[1]

    A. Intensive drill on isolated fricatives, emphasizing the accuracy of articulatory movements, and monitoring for generalization to new words

    B. Extensive ear training exercises with emphasis on the child's ability to judge the accuracy of his own productions and the development of a self-monitoring system

C. Development of a parent-training program with exercise routines to be implemented in the home setting, with the parents providing regular practice on targeted sounds

D. A multifaceted approach combining a synthesized speech system, an analysis of communicatively important targeted words, and practice producing the nearly intelligible words

Record Finish Time _____   **Total Seconds** _____

The answer is (D). The synthesized speech will improve immediate success in a communicative setting, while also providing repeated input of targeted sounds. Using such a system will also facilitate normal language development. The success of the other four alternatives has been limited. Therefore, (A), (B), and (C) are incorrect.

General Timing Strategy

You are given 2.5 hours to complete the Praxis. That is slightly more than 1 minute per question. However, using a full minute is not a good strategy. Rather, it is recommended that you take 48 seconds per question. The rationale for 48 seconds per question is based on a need by most examinees to have a reasonable amount of time to revisit questions answered by guessing and flagged for review. Bear in mind that some short recall questions require as little as 5 seconds. This means that you can take longer than 48 seconds to answer the other lengthy and complex questions.

In a previous chapter it was recommended that questions for which you do not know the answer be flagged and tentatively answered with an educated guess. These are the questions to be revisited when you finish the exam. For the typical examinee,

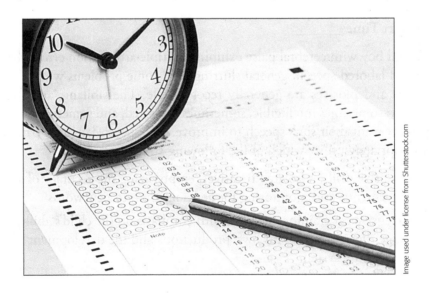

Image used under license from Shutterstock.com

as many as 30 questions might need to be revisited. Therefore, as many as 30 minutes might be needed to revisit these questions.

Setting Your Pace

It is not recommended, nor is it necessary, for you to be conscious of the passing of seconds during the Praxis. Practice, especially with the exercises in this chapter, can instill a habit so pacing becomes automatic. To set the appropriate pace to ensure completion of the Praxis, it will be necessary to establish the proper pace early during the first half-hour. The following is the recommended pacing strategy based on 48 seconds per question as a target.

- Establish a rapid, yet comfortable and efficient pace for the first several questions. Your pace must be comfortable to ensure accuracy. DO NOT SPEED READ the questions. Occasionally monitor the timer and number of questions completed.

- After 15 minutes, check the number of questions completed. You should have completed at least 20 questions. (Remember that the number of questions should be slightly more than the number of minutes lapsed.)

- If you have not reached 20 questions, hasten your speed for short recall questions, carefully avoiding the temptation to speed read. DON'T PANIC. Remember that 48 seconds is an average target. Realize that guessing on unknown questions will save valuable time.

- Continue working for 30 minutes. Check the number of questions answered. You should have completed at least 40 questions.

If you have surpassed this number, this is an excellent pace. If you have not reached 40 questions, mentally diagnose your problem. Realize that you must alter the situation, whatever it is, or risk not being able to return to your flagged questions. Some possible reasons for lack of an appropriate pace include:

- Anxiety
- Boredom/fatigue
- Distraction
- Illness/physical discomfort
- Worry
- Lack of preparation
- Lack of concentration
- Unfamiliarity with the exam format or content
- Slow reading speed
- Indecision

- Poor question attack strategy
- First language interference with reading comprehension
- Tendency to reread questions

Practice and prepare so that these conditions do not apply to you.

Preview Strategy

The preview strategy is a practice for saving time with lengthy questions that have one-word or short phrases as answers. This strategy is useful because it allows a quick view of the answer choices.

The preview strategy is useful with a particular type of question. A typical Praxis question has a lengthy paragraph followed by four answer choices composed of one-word or single-line phrases as in the following examples of answer choices:

A. Hyoglossus

B. Referral for a medical examination

The preview strategy is recommended only for those questions with answer choices composed of one-word or short phrases such as the examples above. The preview strategy is exercised as follows:

- Before completely reading wordy questions, notice whether the set of answer choices is composed of one-word or short phrases.
- Glance quickly at the answer choices only if they are composed of one-word or short phrases. DO NOT READ each answer choice separately.
  - □ If none of the answers are familiar, make a guess and fill in an answer before reading the question.
- If the answer choices are familiar, read them quickly for a sense of the question.
- Return to the question and read it thoroughly.
- If you are certain of the answer, select it without reviewing all the options. Read the other choices and if you need to decide, narrow the choices to two and use reasoning skills to select the best answer.

Single-Letter Strategy

If you run out of time before completing the Praxis, there is an effective strategy for guessing on questions that you might not reach. This strategy requires you to continue working until the final minutes. The single-letter strategy is effective **only** when you have not completed the exam. The single-letter strategy involves marking the same letter for all remaining questions before time elapses as depicted in Figure 8–1 for a written answer sheet. It is important to avoid random selection on the final questions as in Figure 8–2, because random selection decreases your probability of scoring additional points.

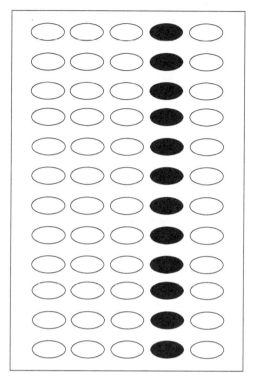

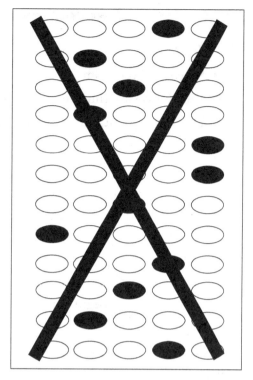

FIGURE 8–1. Single-letter strategy for un-answered questions (Recommended).

FIGURE 8–2. Random marking for unan-swered questions (Not recommended).

You can demonstrate the effectiveness of the single-letter strategy for yourself. Take a sheet of paper and number it 1 through 20. Label it "Sheet #1." In random fashion beside each number write either (A), (B), (C), or (D). Now lay the sheet aside and repeat the procedure on a separate sheet labeled "Sheet #2." Comparing the two sheets, you will probably note that a few letters match by chance. Next choose your favorite letter, either (A), (B), (C), or (D). Now prepare another numbered sheet labeled "Sheet #3" using the same letter for each of the 20 slots so that your answer is the same for each number, as depicted in Figure 8–1. Compare this list to your original Sheet #1 and note the frequency that your letter appears on the original list. Chances are very good that you have more matches between Sheets #1 and #3 than Sheets #1 and #2. Similarly, if you observe the similarities between Figure 8–1 and Figure 8–2 above, you will notice that (D) occurred three out of 12 times. But this is not to suggest that you select (D). You are free to select any letter you desire.

This exercise demonstrates that if you always choose your favorite letter for questions you do not reach, you will probably be correct more often than randomly selecting a letter for each unanswered question. Therefore, remember, if time runs out before you finish, select one letter and select only this letter for all the remaining answers.

Note that the single-letter strategy works only for the unanswered questions you do not reach before time is called. There is no practical value for choosing your favorite letter each time you must take a wild guess as you answer the questions throughout the exam.

Strategies NOT Recommended

Do Not:

- Speed read the exam
- Spend excessive time on difficult questions
- Daydream about other matters
- Interrupt the exam to utilize the facilities unnecessarily
- Allow yourself to be distracted by others
- Take unnecessary and frequent rests
- Read through the answer choices before reading the question for all of the questions
- Leave the exam before time is up for bad reasons
- Stop to recheck the exam if you have not completed all questions
- On rechecking, begin at the first question and review every successive question

Practice the timing strategies with the following set of questions. Use the preview strategy when appropriate.

Record Start Time _____

1. In teaching semantics to a child with a severe language disorder, the words selected by the clinician should be:[2]
   A. Functional in the classroom and home
   B. Functional, developmentally, and environmentally appropriate
   C. Primarily nouns that refer to objects and items in the environment
   D. Phonetically similar to facilitate articulatory movement

2. Which of the following statements best describes congenitally hard of hearing children?[3]
   A. They are usually educated in regular school classes
   B. They have significant impairment of language
   C. They have normal articulation if they use acoustic amplification
   D. They are an extremely heterogeneous

3. A 12-year-old girl shows academic difficulty related to language processing skills. If the child bears a normal range on a performance scale such as the Leiter, Columbia, or Ravens, the speech-language pathologist should presume that:[4]
   A. The child's intellectual development in nonverbal areas is age appropriate

    B. The child's intellectual potential is normal

    C. Some of the child's cognitive skills are age appropriate

    D. The child should be capable of age-appropriate academic achievement in mathematics and logic as long as these subjects are taught nonverbally

4. Analysis of the articulation behavior obtained in assessment is completed for the purpose of:[5]

    A. Determining the cause of the problem

    B. Selecting the target sounds for treatment

    C. Deciding the length of treatment

    D. Determining the relevance of environmental events to the problem

5. Which of the following is not primary to clinical interpretation?[6]

    A. Integration and synthesis of constituent analysis information with clinical testing information

    B. Analyzing the clinical test information

    C. Utilization of knowledge of speech and language disorders apart from that collected from the client

    D. Determination of the accuracy of the clinical hypothesis

6. Which of the following statements concerning ablative surgery of the face, mouth, and pharynx is true?[7]

    A. In most patients receiving this surgery, speech is rendered totally unintelligible

    B. Prosthetic devices may help to restore the normal size and shape of a resonance cavity

    C. Prosthetic devices cannot be used to reclose a resonance chamber

    D. Unilateral nasal excisions will have no effect on nasal resonance as long as the contralateral nasal cavity is undisturbed

7. The best method of designing an effective voice abuse counseling program for an individual client is to:[8]

    A. Present a general list of voice abuses to be eliminated

    B. Ask the client to eliminate selected items in a general list of vocal abuses

    C. Explain the physiologic rationale for eliminating the abuses

    D. Have the client maintain a diary recording the situations, amount of voice use, and rating of the voice to be analyzed for consistent lifestyle patterns related to voice abuse

8. Which of the following areas should be evaluated in the assessment of vocal dysfunction?[9]

    I. Phonatory awareness
    II. Articulatory accuracy
    III. Resonance
    IV. Respiratory function

    A. I, II, and IV only

    B. I, III, and IV only

    C. I, II, and III only

    D. II, III, and IV

9. In evaluating speech and language, baselines are:[10]

    A. Measures of behaviors in the absence of planned intervention

    B. Measures of generalizations of treatment disorders

    C. Measures of maintenance of treated behaviors

    D. Established before the assessment

10. In the evaluation of stuttering, measures of rate:[11]

    A. Are somewhat complicated in that the rate at which words are communicated is not the same as the rate at which fluent speech is produced

    B. Must include both words per minute and syllables per minute

    C. Can be adequately estimated as low, normal, or fast

    D. Need not be taken because therapy always involves reduced rate of speech

11. Neurologic examination of an adult male revealed a left-sided weakness of the arms and lower half of the face. The lesion most likely was located:[12]

    A. In the direct descending motor pathways (pyramidal tract) above the level of the decussation on the left

    B. In the direct descending motor pathways (pyramidal tract) above the level of the decussation on the right

    C. In the direct descending motor pathways (pyramidal tract) below the level of the decussation on the right

    D. In the direct descending motor pathways (pyramidal tract) below the level of the decussation on the left

12. Based on observations of developing stuttering, if a child's stuttering persists, which of the following statements is most accurate?[13]

    A. There is a strong likelihood of change in the characteristics of stuttering as the child matures

    B. Associated or secondary characteristics will occur after puberty

C. All stuttering characteristics will proceed on the same course of development

D. Based on an assessment of the child, the course of future development of stuttering can be predicted

13. All of the following are true with regard to articulation in children with dysarthria except:[14]

A. Children with dyskinetic dysarthria often present with more severe articulation problems than children with spastic dysarthria

B. Articulation error patterns noted in children with dysarthria appear to persist into adulthood

C. Research explicating articulation patterns in children with dysarthria is limited

D. Vowel production is usually not impaired

14. Technically, the treatment of communicative disorders implemented by speech-language pathologists consists of:[15]

A. A strict management of a relation between antecedents, responses, and their consequences

B. Eliminating the neurophysiologic bases of given disorders

C. Enhancing the communicative potential of individuals

D. Removing barriers to social achievement

15. Which of the following is a problem that might be investigated using correlational statistics?

A. A speech pathologist measures the relationship between number of therapy sessions and recovery rate in aphasics

B. A developmental specialist notes the age at which nouns, pronouns, adjectives, and other parts of speech occur in the verbal output of a large group of children

C. An audiologist records the minimal differences between tones detectable by subjects with normal hearing

D. An investigator compares language acquisition patterns in Spanish-speaking and English-speaking children

Time at Finish _____

Compute your timing as follows:

Total Minutes to Completion _____

Total Minutes ÷ (15) (60) = Average Seconds per Question _____

You should have completed this exercise in a maximum of 12 minutes, which is 48 seconds per question. Note how your speed compares.

Answers

1. (B) Communication instruction should reflect the normal developmental process and must also be functional for the child. Thus, (B) is a better answer than (A) or (C). (D) is incorrect because it relates to articulation.

2. (D) Since the statements in (A), (B), and (C) are all characteristic of hearing-impaired children, the best answer is (D) because it reflects the components in all the other choices.

3. (C) The child shows a normal IQ; thus, the cognitive skills measured by the tests show that cognitive skills are age appropriate. Hence (C) is the correct answer. The statements in (A), (B), and (D) are incorrect because they are overgeneralizations of the test results.

4. (B) Assessment is conducted for the purpose of planning for treatment, so (B) is the correct answer. (A), (C), and (D) may be related, but are not the purpose of assessment, so these are incorrect.

5. (B) The question requires the selection of the only false statement. *Primary* is a key word in the question. Clinical interpretation relates to decisions for the outcome of management of disorders. Since analyzing test information is part of the assessment process, it is not primary to interpretation of treatment results. Thus, the correct answer is (B). (A), (C), and (D) are incorrect because they are primary interests in clinical interpretation.

6. (B) The question requires the selection of the only true statement. Prosthetic devices are designed to restore the size and shape of the oral cavity following surgery, so (B) is correct. (A), (C), and (D) are false statements and are incorrect.

7. (D) Maintaining a daily diary will allow the clinician to analyze actual situations for each individual client for direct counseling; therefore, (D) is the correct answer. (A), (B), and (C) are less-effective methods.

8. (B) Articulatory accuracy is not a part of the vocal examination; therefore, any choice containing II is incorrect. The only choice not including II is (B), so it is the correct answer. (A), (C), and (D) are incorrect because they are false statements.

9. (A) Baselines are defined as measurements taken before treatment as a basal of performance to reference progress, so (A) is the correct answer. (B), (C), and (D) are incorrect since these statements do not define baselines.

10. (A) Total rate of communication for stuttering is affected by the rate of fluent speech, as well as the length of the stuttering utterance, so (A) is correct. (B), (C), and (D) are inaccurate statements, so these are incorrect.

11. (B) Before reaching the spinal cord, corticospinal nerve fibers cross to the contralateral side, which influences the side on which clinical signs are seen when a lesion occurs. Since there is weakness on the left side, the lesion was most likely located on the right side. Therefore, the correct answer is (B). (A), (C), and (D) would not characterize left-sided weakness, so they are incorrect.

12. (A) Stuttering symptoms develop and change over time, so (A) is the correct answer since it is the only definite statement. (B) is not always a definite occurrence; therefore, it is an overgeneralization. (C) and (D) are not accurate statements, so these choices are incorrect.

13. (D) The question requires selection of the false statement, which is (D). Since dysarthria results in weakness, decreased muscle tone, decreased range of motion, and abnormal patterns of movement, consonants as well as vowels are affected. (A), (B), and (C) are true statements regarding children with dysarthria.

14. (A) Management of speech and language disorders involves a contingent relation between stimulus variable, target responses, and consequences, so (A) is correct. (B), (C), and (D) are true, but are not incorporated in the correct answer and, therefore, are incorrect.

15. (A) Correlational statistics measure the strength of a relationship between two covarying entities, so (A) is the correct answer. (B) and (D) record the frequency of the variables, and (C) records the differences, so these answers are incorrect.

Frequently Asked Questions

- My timing strategy is to pace myself for one question per minute. I usually have about 15 minutes left, but I know that doesn't leave a lot of time to fix errors. Do you think my strategy is okay?

Your strategy is probably okay, depending on the number of questions you need to review. Using 48 seconds per question, 15 minutes will afford you time to review about 20 questions. But if the questions you need to fix require more reflection, they might take a bit longer than 48 seconds; hence, 15 minutes might not be sufficient.

- When guessing, my strategy is to always mark "C." Is that a good strategy?

When taking a wild guess on any given question, one letter is as good as another. Choosing one letter does not afford any advantage over the long run, so vary your selection. The advantage of the single-letter strategy applies only to the end of the exam when you run out of time.

- Why should we always choose the same letter at the end of the exam?

The reason for marking the same letter is to ensure you get more questions correct. If you mark the questions at random, you decrease your odds of choosing the correct answer. For example, look at the answers for the final 20 questions for the Practice Test Answers in

Appendix A. Count the number of times each letter occurs. You will probably notice that each letter occurs at least twice, but some letters occur more often.

- What is the average length of time to complete the Praxis? Does the average person have enough time to look over their exam at least partially?

The time varies for different examinees and the average is difficult to determine. Typically, there is some time remaining for most examinees. However, most examinees who did not pass reported that they did not finish the exam.

- I know to pick one letter at the end of the exam, but should I use the same letter when randomly guessing in the middle of the exam?

No. Remember, the single-letter strategy is only for questions you do not reach.

- I am having difficulty setting a steady reading pace. I try to read quickly while focusing on details, but I think about how much time I have left and become very anxious. I know that practice will increase speed and accuracy, but is there any other advice?

Take the Practice Test in Appendix A, allowing yourself 2.5 hours. Record your time at the start and finish, but do not exceed the time limit. This should give you a sense of whether your pace is sufficient and relieve your anxiety. If you do not finish in 2.5 hours, take the test again to increase your reading speed using the timing strategies described in this chapter.

- How can I practice answering one question in 48 seconds?

Select 20 consecutive questions in the Practice Test in Appendix A. Set a timer for 15 minutes and complete the 20 questions, noting whether you were able to complete all the questions. Remember, 48 seconds is an average speed. Some questions take as few as 10 seconds.

Sources

1. Educational Testing Service. (1995). *A guide to the Speech-Language Pathology Specialty Area Test* (p. 19). Princeton, NJ: Author.
2. Turton, L. (1982). Communication and language instruction for severely handicapped children and youth. In J. L. Northern (Ed.), *Review manual for speech, language and hearing* (p. 318). Philadelphia, PA: W. B. Saunders.
3. Calvert, D. (1982). Articulation and hearing impairment. In J. L. Northern (Ed.), *Review manual for speech, language and hearing* (p. 232). Philadelphia, PA: W. B. Saunders.
4. Johnston, J. (1982). The language disordered child. In J. L. Northern (Ed.), *Review manual for speech, language and hearing* (p. 286). Philadelphia, PA: W. B. Saunders.
5. McReynolds, L., & Elbert, M. (1982). Articulation disorders of unknown etiology and their remediation. In J. L. Northern (Ed.), *Review manual for speech, language and hearing* (p. 214). Philadelphia, PA: W. B. Saunders.
6. Nation, J. (1982). Management of speech and language disorders. In J. L. Northern (Ed.), *Review manual for speech, language and hearing* (p. 146). Philadelphia, PA: W. B. Saunders.

7. Kuehn, D. (1982). Assessment of resonance disorders. In J. L. Northern (Ed.), *Review manual for speech, language and hearing* (p. 171). Philadelphia, PA: W. B. Saunders.

8. Reed, C. (1989). Voice disorders in the adult. In J. L Northern (Ed.), *Study guide for handbook of speech-language pathology and audiology* (p. 224). Philadelphia, PA: B. C. Decker.

9. Murray, T. (1982). Phonation: Assessment. In J. L. Northern (Ed.), *Review manual for speech, language and hearing* (p. 450). Philadelphia, PA: W. B. Saunders.

10. Johnston, J. (1989). The language disordered child. In J. L Northern (Ed.), *Study guide for handbook of speech-language pathology and audiology* (p. 98). Philadelphia, PA: B. C. Decker.

11. Guyette, T., & Baumgartner, S. (1989). Stuttering in the adult. In J. L. Northern (Ed.), *Study guide for handbook of speech-language pathology and audiology* (p. 168). Philadelphia, PA: B. C. Decker.

12. Thompson, C. (1989). Articulation disorders in the child with neurogenic pathology. In J. L. Northern (Ed.), *Study guide for handbook of speech-language pathology and audiology* (p. 141). Philadelphia, PA: B. C. Decker.

13. Wall, M. (1989). Dysfluency in the child. In J. L. Northern (Ed.), *Study guide for handbook of speech-language pathology and audiology* (p. 160). Philadelphia, PA: B. C. Decker.

14. Op. cit. Thompson, C. (1989). p. 143.

15. Hegde, M. (1989). Principles of management and remediation. In J. L. Northern (Ed.), *Study guide for handbook of speech-language pathology and audiology* (p. 99). Philadelphia: B. C. Decker.

Chapter 9

Guessing Strategies

The test makers of the Praxis encourage guessing to increase performance. Naturally, guessing should not become your general approach to the exam, but should be used when you know something about the question and can select a reasonable choice. Since the Praxis scores only correct answers, blank questions are scored as incorrect. No points are subtracted for wrong answers. Therefore, guessing is likely to increase the number of correct answers. If you know nothing about the question content, take a random guess.

Educated guessing is an essential test-taking strategy. A multiple-choice question is always a game of chance. Since each Praxis question contains four answer choices, even a random guess provides you with a 1 in 4, or 25%, chance of selecting the correct answer. Educated guessing involves increasing this 25% chance to a greater probability. Educated guessing increases the probability of selecting the correct answer depending on the number of choices you are able to eliminate.

There are several effective strategies for guessing on questions for which you know some information. The most effective guessing technique for these questions is avoiding random selection. Random selection of answer choices decreases your probability of scoring additional points. If you have at least some information about the question, use the following strategies to choose among the remaining choices.

Process of Elimination

The reasoning skills discussed in Chapter 4 were designed to assist you in the process of elimination. Recall that reasoning skills are performed on the answer choices that allow you to rule in or rule out particular answers and select the "best" answer. You should understand that the reasoning skills presented in the chapter should not be used as your general approach to the examination. Indeed, if you know the answer automatically, no reasoning skills are necessary. But most Praxis questions are not the type in which the answer is automatic. Therefore, a measure of elimination using the reasoning skills will be necessary.

True/False Strategy

In Chapter 4, the true/false strategy was introduced as a quick method for answering grouping questions and negative stem questions. Recall that this strategy required marking each answer choice with "T" if it is true and "F" if it is false. The correct answer for grouping questions is the choice that contains all of the options marked with "T." For negative stem questions, the correct answer is the single statement marked with "F."

The true/false strategy can also be used for other types of questions to assist in the process of elimination. A variation of the true/false strategy is to use your scratch paper to list A, B, C, and D. As you read through each option, place a check mark beside answer choices that are plausible, and strike through choices that are implausible or otherwise able to be eliminated. This will assist in keeping track of your thoughts, so you won't have to reread each answer choice.

Longest-Answer Strategy

The longest-answer strategy is better than a random guess. Instead of taking a random guess, some examinees opt for the longest answer. This strategy entails choosing the answer choice of greatest length, or the one that makes the best sense and is most complete. Actually, the longest answer strategy is akin to the reasoning ability of predicting the examiner discussed in Chapter 4. A testwise examinee knows that during the construction of a question, the typical item writer might give greater attention and detail when constructing the correct answer, and less attention and detail when constructing the wrong answers. This is indeed the reason why some answer choices are extreme and absurd because the item writer exhausted all plausible options.

The longest answer is the most complete and sensible choice. The longest-answer strategy is most likely to be correct when the answers choices are lengthy sentences, that is, more than one-word or short phrases, such as the example choices presented below with the question omitted.

A. The volume of the external auditory meatus in children is less than that represented by a 2-cc coupler, and consequently the SPL at the tympanic membrane is greater

B. The speech signal will be masked, since room noise with reverberation will be amplified

C. People talk louder to children with hearing aids than adults with hearing aids

D. Measuring hearing loss in children in imprecise and leads to improper fitting[1]

Using the longest-answer strategy, the examinee would select (A), which would be the correct answer.

A word of caution is warranted for the longest-answer strategy. The Praxis test makers are aware and they take care to eliminate such clues to the correct answer. However, you may use the longest-answer strategy in classroom tests with surprising success.

Avoid Extremes

Avoiding extremes among the answer choices is an age-old strategy used widely. Of course, avoiding extremes should be used with reserve when you have some knowledge of the question. It is advisable particularly for taking an educated guess. Avoiding extremes is similar to the reasoning skill of recognition of key words discussed in Chapter 4. When using this strategy, examples of extreme words that should be avoided include:

No

All/All of the above

Not

Never

None/None of the above

Always

Only

Completely

Permanently

Other less extreme words include:

Unimportant

Impossible

Unlikely

Avoiding extremes can sometimes entail eliminating the lowest and highest figure among choices presented in a sequential pattern, as in the example below presented in which the question is omitted.

A. Three

B. Five

C. Six

D. Seven

For this fictitious question, a good guess would be (C). This variation of the strategy entails selecting (B) or (C) while avoiding (A) and (D). Hence, another variation of avoiding extremes is useful rather than taking a random guess.

Avoid Both Opposites

Similar to avoiding extremes, avoiding opposites is often a useful strategy for guessing. It is important to note that avoiding extremes, as all other strategies discussed in this chapter, should only be practiced as a method for guessing, not as a general approach to the exam. When you recognize the correct answer, even if it has an opposite, naturally you should select it and avoid second-guessing your selection, as in the following example.

An investigator is describing the speech of children who have cochlear implants. She finds that the faster the children speak, the less intelligible they are. The investigator obtains a Pearson r correlational relationship with a value of –.92. These results indicate which type of relationship between rate of speech and speech intelligibility?[2]

    A. A strong positive correlational relationship

    B. A strong negative correlational relationship

    C. A canonical correlational relationship

    D. A cause-effect relationship

The answer is (B). Although (A) and (B) are opposites, the correct answer is (B) since the value of r is negative. Since r values range from –1.0 to +1.0, –.92 is a strong negative correlational relationship. (C) and (D) do not characterize the r value, so they are incorrect. For the next example, make an educated guess by using the process of elimination and avoiding extremes.

The neurons that transmit impulses away from the brain are called:[3]

    A. Unipolar neurons

    B. Bipolar neurons

    C. Efferent neurons

    D. Central neurons

The answer is (C). The type of neurons that transmit impulses away from the brain are called *efferent (motor) neurons*, so the correct answer is (C). (A) and (B) are incorrect because they refer to anatomical structure rather than function. (D) is incorrect because it refers to location rather than function.

Avoid Absurd Answers

Absurd answers are not difficult to recognize, especially if they cause you to chuckle. Before selecting your answer, eliminate the absurd answer in the following question.

A graduate student plans to solicit kindergarten children from a public school as participants for thesis research. Before involving the children for the study, the student's ethical responsibility is to:[4]

    A. Obtain written permission from the child, parents, and the school

    B. Inform the parents and the school of the research goals of the project

    C. Ascertain that instructional variables will not bias the results

    D. Make certain that the children are unaware that they are part of a study

The answer is (A). The absurd answer is (D) since it is the ethical responsibility of every investigator to obtain informed consent from all participants, including children. The correct answer is (A) because in the case of children, written permission must be given by legal guardians as well as the institutions charged with the participants' care. (B) and (C) are also incorrect because written permission must be obtained, and (D) is incorrect because participants must be made aware that they are part of a study.

Avoid Negative Statements

Answer choices presented as negative statements are almost always a clue that they should be eliminated. Guess on the following question by eliminating the negative statements.

Pure-tone screening at or below 500 Hz is generally considered inadvisable because:

    A. Hearing tends to fluctuate more at lower frequencies

    B. Most audiometers do not include those frequencies

    C. Thresholds in the lower frequencies are of no diagnostic importance

    D. Ambient noises are more likely to have a masking effect in the lower frequencies

The answer is (D). Environmental noise is likely to interfere with screening at frequencies lower than 500 Hz, so the correct answer is (D). (A), (B), and (C) are incorrect because these statements are inaccurate.

Avoid Unfamiliar Options

This strategy is useful for answers that are composed of one word. When you encounter an option you do not recognize, there is a great probability that it is not the correct answer. An example might be a totally unfamiliar word, syndrome, or condition. There is a natural proclivity for examinees to select this answer when they are unsure of the question content. However, this tendency should be avoided. The next question is an example.

A clinician plans to plot the percentage of correct responses made by a client on treatment probes each day for a period of 3 weeks. This plan accurately describes which of the following?[5]

   A. Before and after research design

   B. Time series design

   C. ABA design

   D. Post hoc design

The answer is (B). A time series design tracks a variable over a period of time using periodic probes, so (B) is the correct answer. A before and after design is a pretest/posttest design, so (A) is incorrect. Similarly, (C) and (D) are incorrect because they do not characterize the plan of the clinician. If you would have chosen (C) because this type of design is unfamiliar to you, your answer would have been incorrect.

A few final words are appropriate on the topic of guessing. It has been emphasized continuously that guessing should not be a general approach to the Praxis. The purpose of guessing is to increase the probability of selecting the correct answer when you are uncertain of the answer. Guessing, in addition to the reasoning skills in Chapter 4, can add points to your score, but these are no substitute for knowledge of the content of the courses. Once you have made a reasonable guess, it is often wise not to change the answer unless you are certain that you are changing to the correct answer. Practice eliminating wrong answers using each of the guessing strategies presented in this chapter in the following exercise.

1. Which of the following statements related to fundamental frequency and intensity is NOT true?

   A. Fundamental frequency and intensity are related to pitch and loudness

   B. Intensity is determined by subglottal air pressure

   C. Fundamental frequency is determined by glottal state and transglottal pressure differential

   D. Fundamental frequency and intensity are related to loudness and pitch, respectively

2. In regard to principles of hearing science, dynamic range refers to:[6]

   A. The full range of frequencies humans can perceive

   B. The decibel range between threshold and the level at which sounds become uncomfortably loud

   C. The decibel range between threshold and the level at which sounds become painful

   D. The decibel range beyond which humans cannot perceive

3. Which of the following are likely to characterize the speech and language of people who are deaf?[7]

I. Omission of /s/ in almost all positions in words
II. Consonant cluster reduction
III. Occasional irrelevance of speech, including nonsequiturs
IV. Improper stress patterns, including excessive pitch inflections
V. A voice that sounds strained and strangled

A. I, II, III, IV

B. I, III, V

C. I, II, IV, V

D. II, III, IV, V

4. A 9-month-old child with a cleft palate has been referred for assessment before surgery. According to genetic history, the child's anomaly can be best explained as a single problem in morphogenesis that led to a cascade of subsequent defects. Which of the following is the most appropriate diagnosis of the child's condition?[8]

A. Fetal alcohol syndrome

B. Apert syndrome

C. Pierre Robin sequence

D. 22q11.2 deletion syndrome

5. A certified clinician in private practice encounters a client who, during a treatment session, discloses statements that reflect suicidal ideation. Which of the following is the most important procedure for the clinician to follow?[9]

A. Tell the client that his life is not all that bad and continue treatment services

B. Refer the client to the appropriate mental health professional

C. Have the client put his plan in writing so she can document the conversation

D. Ignore the statement since it is a mental health issue and not within the clinician's purview

6. A clinician who is a clinical fellow is employed at a rehabilitation company that contracts with a skilled nursing facility. The clinician has received referrals for patients, but few meet the criteria for receiving services. One day, while the clinician was absent from work, her supervisor came to the facility, screened several patients, and left a note for the clinician that the patients will need an evaluation and a plan for treatment. What is the most appropriate option for the clinician?[10]

A. Resign the position because the supervisor is not a good example

B. Review the document left by the supervisor to determine if she agrees with the results and then make a decision

C. Report the supervisor to the Board of Ethics and state licensure board

D. Ask for a meeting with the director of the nursing facility regarding how patient services are provided when she is not present

7. In counseling a client with a speech, language, or hearing disorder, a clinician who is using a client-centered approach will:[11]

   A. Be very direct, making specific recommendations for behavioral changes

   B. Help the client understand conflicts between the id, ego, and superego

   C. Help the client to overcome faulty thinking that is causing distress

   D. Respond with acceptance and empathic listening to both the content and feeling of what the client is saying

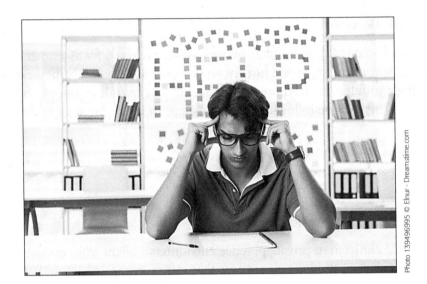

Photo 139496995 © Elnur – Dreamstime.com

Answers

1. (D) The question requires the selection of the false statement. Fundamental frequency is the acoustic correlate of pitch and intensity is the correlate of loudness, so (D) is false, and thus, the correct answer. (A), (B), and (C) are true statements regarding fundamental frequency and pitch, so they are incorrect. The examinee could utilize the true/false strategy to eliminate (A), (B), and (C).

2. (B) The dynamic range is the range between threshold and the point at which sounds become uncomfortably loud; thus, the correct answer is (B). (A) is incorrect because dynamic range does not refer to frequencies. (C) and (D) are incorrect because they do not define dynamic range. When guessing, the examinee could avoid (A) and (D) since they are opposites.

3. (A) Deaf individuals do not typically have a strained or strangled voice, so using the true/false strategy with the Roman numeral choices, statement (V) is false. Therefore, any answer choice containing (V) could be eliminated including (B), (C), and (D).

4. (C) Pierre Robin sequence is a disorder caused by interference in the development of the mandible during gestation in which a single anomaly leads to a cascade of events. Its symptoms include cleft palate, micrognathia, and glossoptosis, so (C) is correct. (A), (B), and (D) are incorrect because their etiologies and symptoms do not characterize those in the question. The examinee could avoid unknown syndromes and eliminate (B) and (D). In addition, a clue to the correct answer (C) is the parallel language of the words *cascade* in the question stem and *sequence* in the correct answer.

5. (C) A referral to the appropriate mental health professional is necessary. Therefore, (C) is the correct answer. The actions expressed in (A), (B), and (D) are contrary to the American Speech-Language-Hearing Association (ASHA) Code of Ethics and thus incorrect. The examinee could eliminate (A), (B), and (D) as absurd answers.

6. (B) The clinician must first determine whether she agrees with the information left by the supervisor and make a determination of whether there is sufficient documentation to proceed with clinical services. Thus, the correct answer is (B). The actions expressed in (A), (C), and (D) are contrary to the ASHA Code of Ethics, and thus incorrect. The examinee could utilize the strategy of avoiding extremes and eliminate (A), (C), and (D).

7. (D) In the client-centered approach, the clinician does not offer advice or give specific recommendations for behavioral changes. Rather, he or she responds with acceptance and empathic listening, so (D) is the correct answer. The statements presented in (A), (B), and (C) are incorrect because they are inconsistent with client-centered counseling. The examinee could use the longest-answer strategy to eliminate (A), (B), and (C).

Frequently Asked Questions

- If you notice earlier than 1 minute before the end of the testing time that you might not finish, should you wait until there is 1 minute left to answer the remaining questions?

Yes. Work to answer as many questions as possible. In the final minute, you should guess using the single-letter strategy discussed in Chapter 8.

- Will 1 minute be sufficient to fill in questions that you might not reach?

If you have more than 20 questions to complete, you will need a lot more time.

- I've heard that there is a magic letter such as B or C when it comes to guessing. Is this true for the Praxis?

Actually, there isn't one magic letter. For a wild guess when you know nothing about the question, I recommend choosing B or C at random because it is a method that avoids extremes. But this is different from the single-letter strategy discussed in Chapter 8.

- For the SAT, I was instructed to guess B or C when in doubt. Is there one letter that is best for guessing for the Praxis?

It is recommended that you choose between B or C only when you must make a random guess, that is, when you know nothing about the question.

- I know you shouldn't change your answer unless you are sure it is incorrect; however, what if you had already guessed the answer in the first place?

Trust your first instinct. Only if you know that you are changing to the right answer should you change your answer.

- I do not guess very well. I have to know the answer to get it right most of the time. Could this potentially affect my Praxis score?

The reasoning skills and strategies in this book are presented to make you a more effective guesser. Your Praxis score should benefit if you use the methods and strategies in this book.

- I know it says to stick to one choice when guessing, but I find that to be unrealistic. Do you think it is smart to alternate guessing answers?

Sticking to one letter every time you guess is a popular myth. Actually, the single-letter strategy is effective only when you run out of time and still have many questions remaining. You should alternate between B and C when you need to make a random guess.

Sources

1. Educational Testing Service. (1995). *A guide to the NTE Audiology Specialty Area Test* (p. 62). Princeton, NJ: Author.
2. Roseberry-McKibbin, C., & Hegde, M. (2006). *An advanced review of speech-language pathology* (p. 650). Austin, TX: Pro-Ed.
3. Ibid. p. 71.
4. Educational Testing Service. (1995). *A guide to the Speech-Language Pathology Specialty Area Test* (p. 114). Princeton, NJ: Author.
5. Ibid. p. 56.
6. Ferraro, J. (2010). Hearing science. In D. Ruscello (Ed.), *Review questions for the Speech-Language Pathology Praxis Examination* (p. 214). Maryland Heights, MO: Mosby/Elsevier.
7. Op. cit. Roseberry-McKibbin, C., & Hegde, M. (2006). p. 557.
8. Vallino, D. (2010). Syndromes and genetics. In D. Ruscello (Ed.), *Review questions for the Speech-Language Pathology Praxis Examination* (p. 300). Maryland Heights, MO: Mosby/Elsevier.
9. Irwin, D. Ethical practices. In D. Ruscello (Ed.), *Review questions for the Speech-Language Pathology Praxis Examination* (p. 323). Maryland Heights, MO: Mosby/Elsevier.
10. Ibid. p. 323.
11. Op. cit. Roseberry-McKibbin, C., & Hegde, M. (2006). p. 693.

Praxis Practice Test

1. Which of the following, if observed in the speech of an African American child, is most likely to represent a dialectal variation rather than an articulation error?

   A. /f/ for /θ/ in postvocalic position
   B. /w/ for /r/ in prevocalic position
   C. /θ/ for /s/ in all positions
   D. Affricates for fricatives in word-final position

2. A 12-year-old native speaker of Spanish who has been studying English as a second language for 3 years is most likely to do which of the following when speaking English in casual conversation with peers at school?

   A. Use the auxiliary "have" in place of "be" in progressive tenses
   B. Use incorrect word order within prepositional phrases
   C. Use conjunctions in place of prepositions
   D. Use multiple negation inappropriately

3. The chewing technique in the treatment of voice disorders is used to accomplish which of the following?

   A. Improve control of loudness
   B. Increase pitch range during voice production
   C. Increase air supply during voice production
   D. Reduce tension in the laryngeal area

4. Intervention for language disorders from a psycholinguistic perspective has been characterized as a facilitation process. The facilitation process is best described by which of the following?

   A. Carrier phrases incorporating new items
   B. Behavior management with a varied-ratio reinforcement schedule
   C. Prepackaged, "canned," or a priori programs
   D. Scaffolding available repertoire and metalinguistic abilities

5. Which of the following is the basic reason for using standardized or normative instruments for assessing language and speech function?

   A. To chart precise increments of change
   B. To provide information for developing specific objectives for therapeutic intervention
   C. To provide a comparison against a standard and to contribute to a database for diagnostic purposes
   D. To describe client and milieu dimensions and to form a database for interaction with the environment

6. Which of the following communication disorders is most frequently associated with significant dysphagia?

   A. Aphasia
   B. Ataxic dysarthria
   C. Flaccid dysarthria
   D. Psychogenic mutism

7. Which of the following is the most reasonable standard to apply when judging whether a client has achieved generalization of a targeted skill?

   A. The client uses the targeted skill in the presence of stimulus conditions not present during the training process and in the absence of reinforcement.
   B. The client no longer needs the clinician to present auditory and/or visual stimuli to elicit the targeted skill.
   C. The client maintains the correct production of the targeted skill when the reinforcement schedule is changed.
   D. The client is able to monitor errors and correct them with only a minimal number of cues from the clinician.

8. The most serious limitation of employing imitation as an intervention strategy for children with a language impairment is that imitation:

   A. Lacks communicative intention
   B. Relies on semantic knowledge
   C. Is clinician controlled
   D. Is contextualized speech

9. Naturalistic teaching chiefly involves which of the following?

   A. Developing complex syntactic structures
   B. Establishing successful and useful communication

   C. Using multiple trials and training techniques
   D. Using more adult-initiated than child-initiated interaction

10. Which of the following is the most common phonological problem later evidenced by children with a history of otitis media during the first 2 years of life?

    A. Velar deviation
    B. Glide deviation
    C. Nasal deviation
    D. Stridency deletion

11. Compared with children who do not have language disorders, children with language disorders tend to:

    A. Take more conversational turns
    B. Initiate topics and direct the flow of conversation more
    C. Ask fewer open-ended questions
    D. Be less deferential and more assertive conversational partners

12. Ms. Badea, a 55-year-old woman with dysphagia, has a delayed swallow reflex. Which of the following is a technique that most often is useful for temporary remediation of her condition?

    A. Cricopharyngeal myotomy
    B. Chin tuck
    C. Thermal stimulation
    D. The Mendelssohn maneuver

13. Of the following, which is generally the most appropriate treatment goal for a client with a laryngectomy?

    A. Production of an esophageal voice
    B. Use of voice prosthesis
    C. Participation in a support group
    D. Restoration of oral communication

14. A 4.5-year-old boy has significant speech and language difficulties exemplified by poor oral-motor control,

slight difficulty in swallowing, high palate, poor tongue mobility, and fasciculation on protrusion. During an evaluation, the speech-language pathologist notes very poor pencil grasp, poor posture, and an inability to complete performance tasks requiring fine motor control. To which of the following should the client be referred in order to obtain additional diagnostic information?

A. A psychologist
B. An otolaryngologist
C. A physical therapist
D. A neurologist

15. Children diagnosed as having specific language impairments are likely to exhibit the greatest deficits in which of the following?

A. Production of sentences with appropriate inflectional morphology and syntax
B. Acquisition of word meanings
C. Comprehension of short sentences
D. Motoric aspects of written expression

16. A third-party reimbursor asks the speech-language pathologist to demonstrate in a diagnostic statement that a child's communication problem is caused by physiological problems. Which of the following observations, if included in the statement, would best satisfy the request?

A. The child's dentition is not yet fully developed but is within normal limits for the child's age.
B. The child has a developmental delay, exhibiting speech that is not age appropriate.
C. The child does not have a functional articulation disorder.
D. The child demonstrates a motor-speech disorder and is unable

to perform voluntarily the oral movements required for speech production.

17. Which of the following is the best example of a functional communication treatment objective?

A. The client will name 80% of the pictures of common objects presented.
B. The client will produce syntactically complete and accurate sentences in a picture-description task.
C. The client will reduce the frequency of occurrence of literal paraphasias to 20% of words produced in spontaneous conversational speech.
D. The client will use the telephone to request assistance in 80% of the appropriate situations presented.

18. Which of the following is the leading cause of neurologic speech and language disorders in adults?

A. Traumatic brain injury
B. Poisoning
C. Neoplasm
D. Cerebrovascular accident

19. A clinician with a master's degree in speech-language pathology is conducting a clinical fellowship as part of the requirements for certification by the American Speech-Language-Hearing Association (ASHA). The clinical fellow developed a language remediation program to be used by school students for carryover and maintenance of skills during the summer months. The clinician plans to organize and implement a 4-week program, using a home office as the site for service delivery. In order to comply with ASHA's ethical and professional

standards, it is most important that the clinician:

A. Have the program approved by a second, more experienced speech-language pathologist.

B. Obtain permission from the local school district supervisor to run the program.

C. Provide weekly updates about the program to the local school district.

D. Work directly under the supervision of a speech-language pathologist who holds ASHA certification and any licensure required by the state.

20. A physician referred a 9-month-old infant who had a low birth weight for an evaluation of development of communication skills. The infant had already passed a neonatal hearing screening. The speech-language pathologist found that the infant followed moving objects visually, and showed interest in mouthing and banging objects, but failed to localize to environmental sounds. In reporting back to the primary care physician, the speech-language pathologist would most appropriately recommend:

A. A psychological evaluation

B. Consideration of auditory amplification

C. Counseling for the parents concerning hearing loss

D. Evaluation of auditory function by an audiologist

21. A speech-language pathologist is planning treatment for a 5-year-old child with multiple speech sound production errors. The most effective strategy for this child would be for the clinician to:

A. Arrange error sounds by developmental pattern and facilitate production for each individual phoneme.

B. Begin with sounds the child can make and use these as bridges to correct production of error sounds.

C. Emphasize auditory discrimination of error sounds from correct sounds.

D. Delineate phonological processes in operation and address them through minimal-contrast pairs.

22. Which of the following statements most accurately describes the comparison of the cognitive problems of children with brain injuries with the cognitive problems of children with learning disabilities?

A. Children with brain injuries tend to require smaller amounts of repetitive teaching and cueing.

B. Children with learning disabilities tend to have poorer social skills.

C. Children with brain injuries tend to have greater difficulty managing their deficits.

D. Children with learning disabilities tend to have greater difficulty with information overload.

23. A correct response rate of 51% on a two-choice picture-pointing task would most likely indicate which of the following?

A. Random pointing response

B. Successful intervention

C. Development of crucial discrimination skills by the clients

D. Readiness to progress to a three-picture pointing task

24. Which of the following is generally considered most effective and appropriate for viewing the vocal folds during phonation?

A. Stroboscopy

B. Endoscopy
C. Fluoroscopy
D. Radiology

25. A clinician who employs an active listening model of counseling is doing which of the following?

A. Responding to both the content and the effect of the client's remarks
B. Listening very carefully and taking extensive notes
C. Conducting a clinician-directed interview
D. Directing the client to specific answers to questions

26. Ms. Martin, aged 69 years, receives speech-language treatment in her home for aphasia secondary to a cerebro-vascular accident (CVA). Medicare is reimbursing the home health care agency for speech-language treatments. In order to ensure that reimburse-ments continue, it is necessary that the speech-language pathologist perform an assessment and write a treatment plan:

A. At least weekly
B. That includes recommendations for family participation in the treatment
C. That is signed by Ms. Martin's physician every 9 weeks as long as treatments are necessary
D. Within 6 months of Ms. Martin's hospitalization for the CVA

27. The presence of language impairment in a child with Down syndrome is often determined by comparing performance on one or more standard-ized language tests with the child's mental age, rather than with the child's chronological age. Although mental age should not be used to specify the need for treatment, mental age can legitimately be used as a performance criterion because:

A. Using chronological age would overidentify language disorders.
B. Using chronological age would underidentify language disorders.
C. Mental age is an error-free measurement.
D. Mental age always correlates with verbal performance.

28. Which of the following types of cerebral palsy is characterized by slow, arrhythmic, writhing, and involuntary movements of extremities?

A. Athetosis
B. Spasticity
C. Hypotonia
D. Rigidity

29. Treatment for apraxia of speech most appropriately emphasizes:

A. Coordination of respiration with phonation and articulation
B. Auditory discrimination, reso-nance, and respiration
C. Auditory-visual stimulation, oral-motor repetition, and phonetic placement
D. Pitch, vocal intensity, vocal quality, and prosody

30. A 32-year-old man is diagnosed as having a moderate fluency disorder. Which of the following, if true for this client, would be the factor indicating the most favorable prognosis for treatment?

A. He received speech therapy when he was in high school.
B. He has recently graduated from college and is preparing for employment.
C. His employer has asked him to seek help for his dysfluency.

D. He considers himself to be mildly dysfluent.

31. Which of the following is NOT a provision of the Health Insurance Portability and Accountability Act (HIPAA)?

    A. Patients may request a copy of their medical records.
    B. Insurance providers may share a patient's medical records.
    C. Health care providers must protect the privacy of medical patients.
    D. Individuals must consent for their medical information to be shared with an insurance agency.

Questions 32–34 are based on the following abstract from a research article:

This investigation was motivated by observations that when persons with dysarthria increase loudness, their speech improves. Some studies have indicated that this improvement may be related to an increase of prosodic variation. Studies have reported an increase of fundamental frequency (F_0) variation with increased loudness, but there has been no examination of the relation of loudness manipulation to specific prosodic variables that are known to aid a listener in parsing out meaningful information. This study examined the relation of vocal loudness production to selected acoustic variables known to inform listeners of phrase and sentence boundaries: specifically, F_0 declination and final-word lengthening. Ten young, healthy women were audio-recorded while they read aloud a paragraph at what each considered normal loudness, twice-normal loudness, and half-normal loudness. Results showed that there was a statistically significant increase of F_0 declination, brought about by a higher resetting of F_0 at the beginning of a sentence and an increase of final-word lengthening from the half-normal loudness condition to the twice-normal loudness condition. These results suggest that when some persons with dysarthria increase loudness, variables related to prosody may change, which in turn contributes to improvement in communicative effectiveness. However, until this procedure is tested with individuals who have dysarthria, it is uncertain whether a similar effect would be observed. (From Watson, P. J., & Hughes, D. [2006]. The relationship of vocal loudness manipulation to prosodic F_0 and durational variables in healthy adults. *Journal of Speech, Language, and Hearing Research, 49*, 636–644.)

32. Which of the following represent the independent variable(s) used in the Watson and Hughes study?

    A. Prosody of dysarthric speech
    B. F_0 declination and final-word lengthening
    C. Vocal loudness
    D. Speech intelligibility and communicative effectiveness

33. Watson and Hughes are cautious when suggesting that the speech of some persons with dysarthria improves due to the prosodic changes that result from increasing vocal loudness. Of the following, which is the most likely reason for this caution?

    A. Only women were studied.
    B. Several acoustic variables related to speech prosody were not included.
    C. The prosody of persons with dysarthria may not show similar loudness effects.
    D. The results were not statistically significant.

34. Which of the following best describes the experimental design of the Watson and Hughes study?

    A. A longitudinal design
    B. A multiple-baseline design

C. A between-subjects design

D. A within-subjects design

35. A 4-year-old child presents the following general speech patterns: liquid gliding, stridency deletion, final consonant deletion, and consonant cluster reduction. Which of the following is the speech-language pathologist's most appropriate recommendation with respect to this child?

   A. Treatment is not needed at this time because the child's speech will improve during the next year.

   B. Treatment should be initiated that focuses on the production of /p/ because it is one of the earliest acquired phonemes.

   C. The child should be referred to a psychologist to rule out cognitive dysfunction.

   D. Treatment should be initiated using a phonological approach focusing initially on the production of final consonants.

36. Immediately following removal of a benign tumor at the base of the brain, a 76-year-old client exhibits severe nasalization and a weak, breathy voice. A 4-month postsurgical assessment reveals no improvement. At this time, the remediation strategy for this client should focus on:

   A. Evaluation for prosthetic and/or surgical intervention

   B. Strengthening exercises for the oral articulators

   C. A trial period using the yawn-sigh technique

   D. Complete vocal rest

37. Which of the following is the ratio of reinforcement that would most quickly cause a newly acquired behavior to become habituated?

   A. Random ratio of tokens to correct responses

   B. Ratio of 1 token to 1 correct response

   C. Ratio of 1 token to 4 correct responses

   D. Ratio of 1 token to 10 correct responses

38. For which of the following conditions is it most appropriate to refer the patient to a prosthodontist for construction of a palatal lift appliance?

   A. Submucous cleft palate

   B. Unrepaired cleft of the secondary palate

   C. Flaccid paralysis of the soft palate

   D. Congenitally short palate

39. Which of the following constitutes the major component of an audiologic rehabilitation program for infants with moderate sensorineural hearing loss?

   A. Development of articulation skills

   B. Development of cognitive skills

   C. Development of social skills

   D. Parent-mediated auditory stimulation

40. A teacher asks the speech-language pathologist for advice regarding a child who talks excessively during class, rarely listens to instructions, and does work only intermittently. Attempts at alternative seating for the child have not been successful. Of the following, which is the most appropriate recommendation that the speech-language pathologist can provide to the teacher?

   A. Reject the idea of sending the child for speech-language therapy because the child seems to speak adequately.

   B. Have the school counselor consider working with the child and the parents on self-control and discipline.

C. Refer the child for evaluation by members of the child-study team.

D. Suggest remedial speech-language services for the child to improve the child's interactive communication.

41. If the goal of a language intervention program for children with language impairments is to facilitate the functional and meaningful use of linguistic forms, then the intervention should:

    A. Focus on comprehension tasks that are at a level immediately above the child's linguistic functioning.

    B. Emphasize the use of pictures showing children's actions rather than adults' actions.

    C. Utilize structured gamelike situations that use imitative tasks.

    D. Present and elicit the linguistic forms in naturalistic contexts.

42. Which of the following is true of the terms *agent* and *subject* as they are used to describe language?

    A. They can be interchanged because both the agent and the subject always agree syntactically with the verb.

    B. They are kept distinct because whether something is an agent depends on semantics, whereas whether something is a subject depends on syntax.

    C. They are kept distinct because it is always possible to determine whether something is a subject, but it is not always possible to determine whether something is an agent.

    D. They are kept distinct because every sentence has an agent but not necessarily a subject.

43. Hearing loss in infants born with cleft palate is usually related to which of the following?

    A. The infant's inability to create positive pressure in the oral cavity

    B. Malformation of the middle ear ossicles associated with malformation of the palate

    C. Eustachian tube dysfunction

    D. Cochlear dysfunction

44. For patients with communication disorders secondary to acquired immune deficiency syndrome (AIDS), the speech-language pathologist would most appropriately:

    A. Provide treatment on a monthly basis.

    B. Provide treatment only as prescribed by the patient's physician.

    C. Avoid physical contact with the patient.

    D. Provide treatment in consultation with the patient's primary-care physician and/or medical team.

45. Which of the following treatment goals related to pragmatics best addresses a young child's use of language?

    A. The child will request a turn, either verbally or through gestures, in a play situation 90% of the time.

    B. The child will produce a two-word combination in a treatment session 90% of the time.

    C. The child will produce correct velars in conversation 90% of the time.

    D. When telling a story, the child will use irregular past tense forms of verbs 90% of the time.

46. A 60-year-old man reports that he has "trouble thinking of names and words" and that this is interfering with his job performance. The problem began after he had a mild cerebrovascular accident, which occurred 3 months earlier. He

does not report any other problems. His conversation is characterized by some hesitancies, latencies, repetitions, interjections, and self-corrections. On the basis of an interview and the results of an aphasia battery, it is concluded that he has a mild aphasia. The most appropriate course of action for the speech-language pathologist is to:

A. Advise the client to wait for three months in order to allow spontaneous recovery to take place.

B. Recommend that the client communicate in writing rather than by speaking in order to accommodate his verbal aphasia.

C. Begin a treatment program designed to decrease dysfluencies in his speech.

D. Implement a treatment program designed to improve word-retrieval skills.

47. Mr. Leone is an 82-year-old man diagnosed with dysphagia. He is fed via a percutaneous endoscopic gastrostomy (PEG) tube because he is at risk for aspiration of thin liquids. From a modified barium swallow study, it was determined that he has laryngeal penetration for nectar-thick liquids in amounts greater than 1 teaspoon. Mr. Leone's daily hydration needs would be best met by:

A. PEG tube primarily

B. Thin liquids perorally in portions of a half teaspoon or less

C. Nectar-thick liquids perorally in portions of a teaspoon or less

D. Honey-thick liquids perorally in portions of a teaspoon or less

48. Which of the following should be the primary focus of early language intervention for at-risk infants?

A. Establishing object permanence through play activities

B. Training primary caregivers to facilitate language learning

C. Introducing the use of augmentative communication

D. Creating readiness activities in the context of play

49. Which of the following is the best action to take initially with a client who exhibits poor oral control of liquids and solids, coughing and choking during feeding, and a history of hospitalization associated with pneumonia?

A. Thicken liquids so the client will be better able to control oral movements for swallowing.

B. Obtain a modified barium-swallow study to determine whether oral feedings are appropriate for the client.

C. Evaluate the client's eating of a variety of foods to determine which foods are safest to eat.

D. Teach the client's caregivers how to control the client's mandibular function while feeding the client.

50. A speech-language pathologist is working with a 30-month-old child who is in the holophrastic stage of linguistic development. The goal of treatment is to facilitate acquisition of complete utterances through play activities. To achieve this goal, the speech-language pathologist can best begin by facilitating the child's:

A. Use of pretend play such as brushing a doll's hair or feeding a doll with a bottle

B. Purposeful exploration of toys

C. Exploration by mouthing or banging of toys

D. Means-end behaviors such as pulling a string to get a toy

51. Ms. Lopez' articulation errors consist of the following: f/v; ʃ/dʒ; and s/z. On the basis of these errors, the speech-language pathologist would most appropriately begin remediation that focuses on:

    A. Manner
    B. Place
    C. Fricatives
    D. Voicing

52. Ms. Helene, a 60-year-old woman with a suspected neurological disorder, is referred for speech-language evaluation. She achieves a score of 35/50 on a measure of confrontation object-naming ability. This score is below norms established for individuals of her age and educational level. Based on these results alone, which of the following statements can most reliably be made about Ms. Helene's disorder?

    A. She has aphasia, but the type of aphasia cannot be specified on the basis of this test score.
    B. She does not have aphasia but probably does have a memory disturbance.
    C. She probably has visual-perceptual deficits, but this should be confirmed by specific visual-perceptual testing.
    D. She has difficulty with naming, but the precise nature of the deficit cannot be determined on the basis of this test score.

53. Exposure of several hours to continuous music with an overall level of 100 dB SPL at a live concert will most likely produce:

    A. Tinnitus and a temporary threshold shift in the high frequencies
    B. Tinnitus and a decrease in speech perception

    C. Temporary threshold shift in the low frequencies
    D. Permanent threshold shift

54. A 6-year-old client who is a bilingual English-Spanish speaker produced the following statements during a speech-language assessment:

    > I cutted my finger.
    > I played with her yesterday.
    > She eated too much candy.
    > You like ice cream?
    > Maria is going?
    > Father is happy. Buy a new car.

    Based on the sample, the speech-language pathologist should initiate treatment by focusing on which of the following?

    A. Adjectives and imperatives
    B. Irregular verbs
    C. Prepositional phrases
    D. Conjunctions and embedding

55. Mr. Charles, age 78, was diagnosed with Alzheimer's 9 years ago. A recent speech and language evaluation at his nursing home indicated severe deficits in verbal reasoning, memory, word finding, discourse, pragmatics, phonology, semantics, and syntax. Which of the following would be the most appropriate course of treatment for the speech-language pathologist?

    A. Individual treatment to improve his receptive and expressive language skills beginning with the areas in which he is least deficient
    B. Individual treatment to improve his receptive and expressive language skills beginning with the areas in which he is most deficient
    C. Individual treatment to improve verbal memory and auditory processing skills before attempting to remediate the linguistic deficits

D. Examine living conditions and, if necessary, educate the nursing staff concerning the nature of his deficits and strategies to help him communicate

56. A public-school speech-language pathologist is employed in a state that sets the maximum caseload at 35. However, this clinician's caseload is currently at 34 with a waiting list of 10 additional students. The school principal insists that the speech-language pathologist enroll these 10 students immediately because the district cannot locate another clinician to assist with the caseload. Which of the following is the most appropriate strategy for the speech-language pathologist to implement to address this situation?

A. Enroll the 10 students and provide the principal with a written statement mentioning the number, frequency and type of treatment needed by the students.
B. Refer the 10 students to a speech-language pathologist working in a private setting.
C. Suggest that the principal ask a school speech-language pathologist from another school district to take the 10 students.
D. Maintain the current caseload until an additional speech-language pathologist is hired.

57. Linguistic approaches to treatment of sound production errors are based on the notion that the errors are systematic and rule-based and that the goal of treatment is to modify a child's rule system to approximate the rule system used by adults. Which of the following is a statement of a treatment goal that reflects a linguistic approach?

A. The child will contrast alveolar stops with velar stops in meaningful word pairs.
B. The child will produce voiceless alveolar sibilants correctly in unstructured conversation.
C. The child will coarticulate stop plus liquid clusters.
D. The child will produce [r] in isolation without lip rounding.

58. In a test instrument for expressive morphology for children with grammatical disorders, the items require the examinee to identify sentences containing grammatical errors. The purpose of the test is to determine whether the examinee is acquiring rules of morphology and syntax that are appropriate for age and sociocultural dialect. For nonbiased assessment of speakers of African-American English, which of the following items would impose an unfair penalty if scored as incorrect for these speakers?

A. We wented home
B. He no want none
C. She drop she glasses
D. We seen him running

59. A 42-year-old client with upper-extremity and lower-extremity weakness and a diagnosis of amyotrophic lateral sclerosis is referred for a speech-language evaluation. The evaluation reveals a progressive severe dysarthria that is characterized by imprecise articulation secondary to bilateral facial and lingual weakness, atrophy, and fasciculations; mild to moderate hypernasality and weak pressure consonants with associated nasal emission during speech; and strained/harsh/groaning voice quality with occasional inhalatory stridor.

Speech intelligibility is poor. Which of the following will most effectively improve this client's ability to communicate?

A. Teflon injection into one or both vocal folds
B. Palatal-lift prosthesis
C. Pharyngeal flap
D. Augmentative communication system

60. Language intervention for a child at the one-word stage should be most strongly influenced by a consideration of the child's:

A. Motor skills
B. Cognitive skills
C. Syntactic skills
D. Articulation skills

61. Computer software that has been developed to facilitate speech and language treatment can best be used:

A. In group sessions when the speech-language pathologist's caseload precludes working individually with clients
B. By clients in place of services that would otherwise be provided by a speech-language pathologist
C. By clients under the direction of speech-language pathologists
D. When the client refuses to communicate with the speech-language pathologist

62. An adult client exhibits visuospatial disorganization, an inability to initiate interactions, unilateral neglect, and lack of facial expression. This combination of behaviors is most accurately associated with which of the following?

A. Right-hemisphere brain injury
B. Left-hemisphere cerebrovascular accident

C. Bilateral traumatic brain injury
D. Alzheimer's dementia

63. Two months after undergoing surgery to improve velopharyngeal function, a client continues to exhibit nasal airflow and articulatory compensations in production of pressure consonants. The speech-language pathologist would most appropriately:

A. Refer for consideration of prosthetic management
B. Request a nasoendoscopic study
C. Inform the surgeon that the client is not making satisfactory progress
D. Provide speech treatment

64. To justify the provision of treatment for a 2.5-year-old child with apraxia of speech, which of the following would be LEAST important for the speech-language pathologist to include in the evaluation report?

A. A description of the child's typical communication with peers
B. Relevant prognostic data
C. Information about apraxia of speech
D. A description of the language development of the child's older siblings

65. A 4-year-old girl with dysfluency is referred for a speech and language assessment. In deciding whether she is displaying typical nonfluent behavior rather than stuttering, the speech-language pathologist would appropriately assign greatest importance to which of the following?

A. The length of time she has been dysfluent
B. The amount of communication during the assessment
C. The rate at which she talks
D. The nature and frequency of her dysfluent behaviors

66. Establishment of which of the following is most important in ensuring the results of any diagnostic test of speech or language are replicable?
    A. Age norms for the test
    B. Content validity
    C. Interjudge reliability
    D. Split-half reliability

67. Intervention from a speech-language pathologist for a nursing home resident who is in a late state of progressive dementia would most effectively focus on:
    A. Conversational intelligibility
    B. Recall of salient vocabulary words
    C. Comprehension of social discourse
    D. Assisting in communication routines

68. Control over the fundamental frequency of the laryngeal tone is most closely related to the activity of which of the following muscles?
    A. Posterior cricoarytenoid
    B. Lateral cricoarytenoid
    C. Cricothryoid
    D. Hyoglossus

69. Which of the following procedures would be effective in remediating a falsetto voice for an adult male with a severe bilateral hearing loss?
    A. Development of phonation from coughing
    B. Pushing exercises
    C. Auditory training
    D. Manual depression of the larynx

70. Excessive nasality is associated with insufficient palatal closure. Which of the following is the easiest way for a speaker to determine whether there is inappropriate nasal airflow?
    A. Looking in a mirror while speaking
    B. Holding a feather in front of the mouth while speaking
    C. Being aware of vowel-sound productions
    D. Speaking while alternately leaving the nostrils open and pinching them closed

71. A speech-language pathologist is having an initial consultation with a self-referred adult with a fluency disorder. The client had been enrolled in treatment programs with this clinician five times before. The client had reached 90% fluency during the previous treatment sessions but discontinued treatment. The client currently exhibits 60% fluency with motoric secondary characteristics. The client does not maintain normal eye contact and engages in few interpersonal interactions. The speech-language pathologist would most appropriately:
    A. Encourage the client to re-enroll for treatment services.
    B. Encourage the client to take responsibility for maintaining fluency by using techniques learned in the previous treatment sessions.
    C. Recommend that the client schedule a neurological evaluation.
    D. Refer the client for psychological counseling.

72. Which of the following is NOT useful for the assessment of swallowing ability?
    A. Videofluoroscopy
    B. Bedside evaluation
    C. Fiberoptic endoscopy
    D. Gastrostomy

73. Speech-language pathologists often have a responsibility to communicate with the parents of children with severe disabilities. In terms of mourning theory, when would parents normally be most receptive to information

and advice provided by professionals regarding their child?

A. During the mourning period, when the mother and newborn are dismissed from the hospital

B. When the parents are working through their feelings about the child's disabilities

C. When the parents fully realize the extent of the child's disabilities and the limitations of treatment and education

D. During the recovery period, when the parents have acquired greater confidence in their capacity to care for the child and greater motivation to cope with the child's disabilities

74. Individuals diagnosed as having hemifacial microsomia are also most likely to have:

A. Laryngeal dysfunction
B. Protrusive mandible
C. Ear malformation
D. Webbed fingers or toes

75. A child repeatedly inserts an inappropriate sound in specific environments in monosyllabic words; for example, [k j ʌ p] for [k ʌ p]. Which of the following would likely be most helpful for this child as a target for treatment?

A. Words important in the child's environment, including the names of favorite toys, close friends, and familiar places

B. Bisyllabic words for which a minimal-contrast pair can be easily identified

C. Words containing phonemes that have distinctive features in common with the sound the child inserts inappropriately

D. Words containing combinations of phonemes that are similar in place and manner to those into which

the child makes the inappropriate insertion

Questions 76–79 refer to the following case:

Michael is a 32-month-old boy who has been receiving intervention services for over the past 10 months for delayed speech and expressive language development. Although his birth was reportedly unremarkable, Michael has a history of recurrent otitis media with effusion. His parents describe him as a "well-behaved and quiet boy." When Michael began receiving services, he communicated mainly through gestures and crude vocalizations. An open resting mouth position with slight tongue protrusion was sometimes noted. However, his receptive language skills were found to be age appropriate and he showed no oral motor deficits during feeding. Michael's expressive language skills have shown some progress since he began working with the speech-language pathologist, but he remains poorly intelligible. Michael's imitation of tongue, lip, and jaw movements is characterized by inconsistent groping and errors of sequencing not observed in his spontaneous oral movements. Michael has an age-appropriate vocabulary and he produces utterances of three words. Articulation errors, especially metathesis of phonemes and syllables, increase as his utterance length increases. Michael's intelligibility is greatest at the single-word level. Automatic speech and highly familiar utterances are much more intelligible than his imitated productions.

76. As a part of ongoing assessment, the speech-language pathologist's most appropriate action is to have Michael's parents consult with his primary care provider for referral to:

A. A special educator
B. A neurologist
C. A psychologist
D. An otolaryngologist

77. Michael shows the speech behaviors that are typical of children diagnosed with which of the following?
    A. Developmental apraxia of speech
    B. Conductive hearing loss
    C. Hyperkinetic dysarthria
    D. Specific language impairment

78. Based on Michael's case history, the speech-language pathologist would most appropriately provide activities to:
    A. Stabilize muscle tone to improve gross motor support of speech movement
    B. Improve receptive language ability
    C. Strengthen tongue, lip, and jaw muscles
    D. Increase the accuracy of CV, VC, and CVC syllable sequences

79. Given Michael's age, which of the following is likely to be the most effective strategy for speech and language intervention?
    A. Using structured play to address short-term goals
    B. Facilitating Michael's ability to self-monitor his speech
    C. Instructing Michael's parents in structured home exercises for their son
    D. Discontinuing services until Michael reaches school age

80. Most state laws regarding freedom of access to information stipulate that client records kept or written by health care professionals can be:
    A. Reviewed only by other health care professionals
    B. Reviewed only by the clients themselves unless the client provides written per to share with others
    C. Reviewed by anyone who submits a formal written request
    D. Released only by subpoena

81. It is most appropriate for the speech-language pathologist to treat hyperadduction of the vocal folds by having the client:
    A. Increase muscular effort through pushing or lifting while vocalizing
    B. Use light and gentle vocal fold contacts
    C. Attempt quick onset of phonation
    D. Use drills with exaggerated contrastive stress on words

82. Which of the following errors is likely to persist the longest in the speech of children who are learning Standard American English (SAE) as a first language and are following the normal developmental course for speech and language acquisition?
    A. Assimilation
    B. Consonant cluster reduction
    C. Final-consonant deletion
    D. Stopping

83. Which of the following is an accurate statement about whispered speech?
    A. It is produced by approximating the arytenoid cartilages so that their medial surfaces are in direct contact.
    B. Its fundamental frequency is typically specifiable at between 60 and 80 Hz.
    C. It is composed largely of aperiodic sounds.
    D. Spectrographic analysis of it reveals no discernible formants for the vowels.

84. Of the following sentences, which represents the greatest degree of syntactic complexity?
    A. Is John helping Bill?
    B. Why isn't John helping Bill?
    C. John isn't helping Bill.
    D. John is helping Bill.

85. A 5-year-old girl with a repaired cleft palate has recently undergone a pharyngeal flap operation to correct velopharyngeal incompetence but she continues to use glottal stops, pharyngeal fricatives, and mid-dorsum palatal stops. Which of the following would be the most appropriate course of action for the speech-language pathologist to assume?

    A. Recommend that the child be examined by a cleft palate team to determine the cause of the persistent articulation errors.
    B. Refer the child back to the surgeon to determine the need for a revision of the pharyngeal flap.
    C. Initiate articulation treatment to teach the correct placement of the stops and fricatives.
    D. Initiate voice treatment to teach a soft glottal attack.

86. A 4-year-old child exhibits the following production errors.

    w/r θ/s t/ʃ t/tʃ z/dʒ t/k d/g

    If a target sound for initial intervention were to be selected on the basis of established developmental norms, that sound would be:

    A. /r/
    B. /s/
    C. /ʃ/
    D. /k/

87. A speech-language pathologist sees a college-educated 22-year-old man who has sustained a brain injury as the result of a motor vehicle accident 18 months earlier. The man was unconscious for 5 days and had post-traumatic amnesia for 3 months. In the last year he has held three unskilled jobs, from which he was released for unspecified reasons. On the basis of this information only, the most pervasive condition in this case is likely to be impaired:

    A. Visual construction
    B. Attention and memory
    C. Praxis
    D. Speech

88. A speech-language pathologist evaluated a 5-year-old boy presenting with microcephaly, microdontia, and limited joint movement. The child was friendly and talkative and used good syntax, but he displayed some perseveration when using colloquial expressions. The speech-language pathologist's may most appropriately conclude that the child:

    A. Has a possible self-concept problem due to his appearance but is trying hard to be sociable; therefore, he should be encouraged to interact more with peers
    B. Might be exhibiting symptoms of Williams syndrome; therefore, he should receive a cognitive evaluation, and his family should be given genetic counseling
    C. Is exhibiting characteristics of a chromosomal syndrome and as such may be cognitively impaired; and should be referred for a neurological evaluation and a review of the case by a physical therapist
    D. Most likely has Marshall syndrome requiring further evaluation using a team approach including a physical therapist and audiologist

89. Cognitive therapy for stuttering focuses on which of the following?

    A. Extinguishing the overt, dysfluent speech behavior by withholding positive reinforcement
    B. Changing faulty beliefs about self-control and the perceived benefits of stuttering

C. Changing handedness when use of the right hand was forced on a left-handed person

D. Providing positive reinforcement during periods of fluent speech

90. Successful use of an alternative/ augmentative communication system is based on factors such as selecting appropriate vocabulary, seating and positioning, and having a reliable method of controlling the system. To facilitate the most effective use of the system, clinicians most often advocate which of the following approaches?

A. Unimodal
B. Multimodal
C. Bimodal
D. Vocal

91. A physician advised the spouse of a client that melodic intonation therapy (MIT) would improve the client's speech considerably. The most appropriate next action by the speech-language pathologist would be to:

A. Provide MIT as recommended
B. Refuse to provide MIT
C. Discuss with the physician the inappropriateness of a physician's making recommendations for speech treatment
D. Consider the potential value of incorporating MIT into the client's treatment

92. In the treatment of acute Wernicke's aphasia, the initial focus should be upon:

A. Encouraging self-monitoring of the adequacy of verbal output
B. Encouraging the client to sing
C. Improving the client's ability to elaborate verbally
D. Increasing the complexity of sentence structure

93. A prospective client is described as a man in his forties who is under chronic stress. He uses his voice extensively in daily life and exhibits glottal fry. He has a tense, aggressive personality. This description is a classic profile of a person at high risk for:

A. Spastic dysphonia
B. Ventricular dysphonia
C. Acute laryngitis
D. Contact ulcers

94. Which of the following is a typical symptom observed in cases of cerebellar involvement?

A. Overshooting or undershooting an intended action
B. Rigidity during voluntary motions
C. Spasticity during involuntary action
D. Word-finding difficulty

95. Which of the following would be most likely to help a client who has aphonia?

A. Development of phonation through coughing or throat clearing
B. Development of hard glottal attack
C. Pairing the production of /s/ and /z/
D. Easy initiation of phonation

96. When counseling the parents of a child who has an articulation disorder, the speech-language pathologist would cite developmental norms to show which of the following?

A. The child's misarticulation will interfere with reading skills.
B. A percentage of children of a similar age can correctly articulate the misarticulated sound.
C. The misarticulated sound is not a frequently occurring sound in the language.
D. The misarticulation is caused by faulty learning.

97. If a child's language exhibits the phonological process of gliding, the child might say "wed" for "red." When asked, "Do you mean wed?," the child may respond, "No, wed!" Such a response demonstrates which of the following?

A. Phonological development lags behind semantic development.
B. Semantic development lags behind phonological development.
C. Linguistic competence lags behind linguistic performance.
D. Linguistic performance lags behind linguistic competence.

98. Which of the following would provide the most important diagnostic information when a speech-language pathologist is making a differential diagnosis between developmental apraxia of speech and flaccid dysarthria in a child?

A. A history of the child's development of chewing, eating, and swallowing
B. A history of the child's language development
C. A history of the child's middle ear pathology
D. The child's willingness to function in sociocommunicative events

99. Which of the following most accurately describes the etiology of cleft palate?

A. Genetic syndrome alone
B. Environmental influences alone
C. Genetic factors interacting with environmental influences
D. The mother's consumption of alcohol during pregnancy

100. Speakers of a language possess metalinguistic abilities that provide insight into their linguistic competence. Sentences such as "Visiting friends can be a nuisance" are especially useful to test an individual's ability to:

A. Distinguish sentences from nonsentences
B. Recognize syntactic ambiguity
C. Interpret metaphorical language
D. Distinguish homonyms by means of syntactic cues

101. Prostheses such as those developed by Blom-Singer or Panje help the client with laryngectomy to produce sound by:

A. Pushing air in blasts from the lungs
B. Shunting air from the trachea to the esophagus to be used like esophageal speech
C. Keeping liquids and food particles out of the trachea by valve action
D. Venting excess air from the trachea to reduce interfering stoma noise

102. Following anoxic encephalopathy, an individual is likely to experience the most significant long-term impairments in the area of:

A. Prosody
B. Dysphagia
C. Resonance
D. Memory

103. A 55-year-old woman, recently hospitalized for cerebrovascular accident (CVA), is referred for evaluation of "stuttered speech." The initial conversation with the client indicates that speech is characterized by frequent initial phoneme repetitions and prolongations with associated mildly effortful eye blinking. Which of the following pieces of information is crucial to accurate speech diagnosis and decisions regarding management of the speech problem?

A. The site and extent of the lesion associated with the suspected CVA

B. The handedness of the client and that of her first-degree relatives

C. Whether the client has any associated dysphagia or dysphonia

D. Whether the dysfluency occurred before or after the CVA

104. A number of research reports have described poor auditory memory in children with language impairments. Which of the following can most appropriately be concluded from these studies?

A. Poor auditory memory can be improved by language intervention programs that focus on teaching vocabulary and word meanings.

B. Poor auditory memory is a reflection of a language impairment, and clinicians cannot foster improvement.

C. Poor auditory memory could be a reflection or a cause of a language impairment or could be related to some other factor, and further research is needed.

D. All children with language impairments should be tested for auditory memory because auditory memory is good prognostic indicator.

105. When providing treatment to a client who is using an electronic augmentative communication device, the speech-language pathologist's primary goal should be to:

A. Ensure that the client develops skill in using every technical aspect of the device.

B. Ensure that caregivers learn how to modify the hardware and software to meet the client's communication needs.

C. Train the client to use the device independently and interactively in a variety of settings.

D. Help the client develop the skills necessary for moving to a more sophisticated device.

106. Which of the following is a type of perturbation that can be measured to determine the amount of noise in the voice?

A. Changes in the frequency range between F_0 and F_1 over time

B. Changes in the frequency range between F_1 and F_2 over time

C. Changes in the frequency range between F_2 and F_3 over time

D. F_0 cycle-to-cycle variations in period over time

107. A videofluorosopic study of a client with dysphagia revealed pooling of liquids in the valleculae. Which of the following is the most likely overt symptom the client will experience?

A. Watery eyes during swallowing

B. Oral pocketing of foods

C. Coughing after swallowing

D. Neuralgia

108. A 1-year-old girl was observed during a speech-language evaluation. To express herself, the child occasionally touched her mother, gained eye contact, and then gestured toward an object. If the child's overall development is normal, within the next month the child will begin to:

A. Use consistent sound and intonation patterns for specific intentions

B. Reach for objects she desires

C. Establish joint reference with her mother

D. Use recognizable words and phrases to express her intentions

109. Performing which of the following would likely yield the most useful

information about the effectiveness of an intervention strategy?

A. Comparing the results to performance on standardized assessment instruments

B. Using a single-case design (ABAB) comparing baseline performance to treatment performance

C. Utilizing a subjective-objective assessment plan (SOAP)

D. Developing specific pretests to use before treatment

110. Primary motor innervation to the larynx and velum is provided by which cranial nerve?

A. Vth
B. VIIth
C. IXth
D. Xth

111. The major objective of auditory training of a client with a hearing loss is to:

A. Improve the client's awareness of position and movements of the speech mechanism.

B. Improve the client's kinesthetic and auditory awareness.

C. Increase the client's kinesthetic and proprioceptive discrimination.

D. Teach the client to make visual discriminations among speech sounds.

112. Which of the following is the most accurate description of the likely effects on a young child of repeated episodes of otitis media with intermittent hearing loss?

A. There is no effect on syntactic development.

B. There is a limited effect on phonological development.

C. There is a mild to moderate effect on phonological development.

D. There is a mild to moderate effect on overall language development.

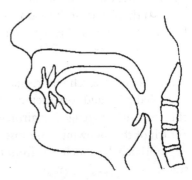

113. An individual is attempting to sustain /f/ as shown in the midsagittal view above. The most important reason why this speaker will not produce an acceptable /f/ is that:

A. The upper central incisors are tipped too far labially.

B. The low central incisors are tipped too far labially.

C. Intraoral air pressure will be insufficient.

D. Lip placement is inadequate.

114. An otolaryngologist has referred a 45-year-old man for voice treatment following medialization thyroplasty for a paralyzed vocal fold. Of the following, which is the most appropriate treatment strategy for the speech-language pathologist to implement?

A. Assist the client to produce a soft glottal attack.

B. Digital manipulation of the client's neck to reduce-strap muscle tension.

C. Assist the client to produce a hard glottal attack.

D. Employ techniques aimed at increasing speech airflow.

115. To provide greater independence for a client with a brain injury in a late stage of speech-language treatment, which

of the following techniques is most appropriate?

A. Increasing memory retention span
B. Copying geometric forms
C. Using word-repetition drills
D. Teaching compensatory strategies

116. According to research on the development of Brown's morphemes in young children, which of the following is a determinant of acquisition order?

A. Frequency of use in adult speech
B. Phonological ease of production
C. Figurative language ability
D. Semantic and syntactic complexity

117. A speech and hearing clinic has recently opened, but referrals are slow in coming. Which of the following would be most appropriate and effective for the clinic's director to do first?

A. Ask local hospitals to provide names of recent clients likely to need speech-language services.
B. Identify and define the major consumer groups and referral sources and develop a plan to reach them.
C. Identify the weaknesses in the competition, and inform consumer groups and referral sources of the weaknesses.
D. Wait for demand to increase on its own, because marketing speech and language services is against the ASHA Code of Ethics.

118. A client with anomic aphasia is a native speaker of Spanish with fair proficiency in English. Production of the word "shoes" as [tʃ u z] on a repetition task is most likely due to which of the following factors?

A. Phonological interference from the speaker's native language
B. Semantic interference from the speaker's native language

C. Semantic paraphasia due to the aphasia
D. Phonemic paraphasia due to the aphasia

119. A child with discourse problems is most likely to require remediation directed at which of the following?

A. Morphology
B. Instrumental language
C. An initial lexicon
D. Cohesive devices

120. Research regarding the use of intensive phonemic awareness treatment for children who have difficulty learning to read has demonstrated that the training:

A. Is effective mainly with children who have remediated all phonological process errors
B. Is effective only when combined with a supplemental literacy program
C. Also improves oral discourse ability
D. Might have no relationship to improved reading ability

121. The speech reception threshold (SRT) is a basic component of an evaluation of hearing function. Which of the following statements about the SRT is most accurate?

A. It is measured in decibels and corresponds to the intensity level at which spondaic words can be recognized approximately 50% of the time.
B. It is more difficult to administer than pure-tone audiometry because of the nature of the acoustic signals.
C. It makes use of test materials that are limited to monosyllabic words.
D. It provides information on how well speech is understood at conversational levels.

Questions 122–123 refer to the following audiogram:

PURE TONE AUDIOGRAM

Frequency in Hertz

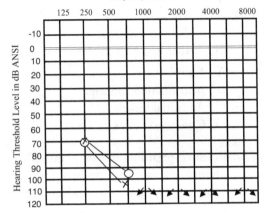

122. Which of the following will characterize the speech of the individual whose audiogram is depicted in the audiogram above?

   A. Slurred speech that is unintelligible
   B. Misarticulations of consonants with vowel integrity
   C. Misarticulation of most consonants and vowels with poor pitch control
   D. Excessive loudness

123. The type of hearing loss characterized by the audiogram is:

   A. Moderate
   B. Profound
   C. Severe
   D. Severe to profound

124. In the perception of speech sounds, which formants are most useful for recognition of vowels sounds?

   A. F_1, F_2, and F_3
   B. F_1 and F_2
   C. F_2 and F_3
   D. F_1 and F_3

125. An infarct sustained in which of the following locations would result

in difficulty in comprehension of language?

   A. Wernicke's area
   B. Frontal lobe
   C. Broca's area
   D. Prefrontal area

126. Which of the following is LEAST related to vocal intensity?

   A. Constriction of the oral cavity
   B. Lung capacity
   C. Vocal fold constriction
   D. Raising of pitch

127. A condition characterized by random, involuntary uncoordinated muscle contractions and jerks is known as:

   A. Athetosis
   B. Chorea
   C. Ballism
   D. Tourette's syndrome

128. Differential diagnosis of apraxia of speech from dysarthria is confirmed by:

   A. Presence of articulatory errors
   B. Presence of prosodic deficits
   C. Neurological soft signs
   D. Diminished muscle strength

129. A clinician suspects that a child has a mild learning disability. The clinician decides to test her theory by assembling tasks that are immediately above the child's estimated developmental level and that examine the child's ability to complete the tasks. This is followed by treatment and re-examination following the treatment sessions. The clinician's approach to assessment is known as:

   A. Dynamic assessment
   B. Functional assessment
   C. Portfolio assessment
   D. Authentic assessment

130. Which of the following extrinsic
     muscles is primarily responsible for
     protrusion of the tongue?
     A. Hyoglossus
     B. Palatoglossus
     C. Genioglossus
     D. Styloglossus

131. The symptoms of traumatic brain
     injury are the result of damage to
     which area of the brain?
     A. Frontal lobe
     B. Parietal lobe

C. Diffuse areas
D. Localized sites

132. In the production of voice at the
     laryngeal level, rotation and rocking
     movements of the vocal folds are
     accomplished by:
     A. Cricoarytenoid joint
     B. Thyroid cartilage
     C. Arytenoid cartilages
     D. Cricoarytenoid and cricothyroid
        joint

Sources

Questions 1 to 31 from Educational Testing Service (2006, May 25). *The Praxis Series Test Code 0330: Speech-language pathology practice questions* (Chapter 5, pp. 47–53).

Questions 35 to 75 from Educational Testing Service (2006, May 25). *The Praxis Series Test Code 0330: Speech-language pathology practice questions* (Chapter 5, pp. 54–65).

Questions 80 to 121 from Educational Testing Service (2006, May 25). *The Praxis Series Test Code 0330: Speech-language pathology practice questions* (Chapter 5, pp. 65–74).

Praxis Practice Test Answers and Explanations

1. **(A)** The use of voiceless labiodental fricatives for voiceless interdental fricatives (e.g., /f/ for /θ/) is a feature of African-American English (AAE), so (A) is the correct answer. (B) and (C) identify developmental errors that are not peculiar to AAE, so those answer choices are incorrect. (D) is incorrect because the use of affricates for fricatives in word-final position is a type of stopping that is not characteristic of AAE and is more likely to be a developmental error if it occurs.

2. **(D)** Multiple negation is a grammatical feature of Spanish, but not of Standard English. Thus, the two languages contrast in this respect. Multiple negation could persist as a speaker attempts to learn Standard English through a phenomenon known as fossilization which is common in accented speech. In Spanish, the sentence "I didn't tell him anything" might be rendered as "No le dije nada." The literal translation of this sentence is "I didn't tell him nothing." (D) is, therefore, the correct answer. (A) is incorrect because the progressive aspect is produced similarly in Spanish and

English. (B) and (C) are incorrect because the structure of prepositional phrases and the use of conjunctions are similar in both languages.

3. **(D)** The chewing technique is used to reduce muscular tension in the laryngeal area, so (D) is the correct answer. (A) and (C) are incorrect because the control of loudness and an increase in air supply require increased muscular tension in the respiratory system and thus, are accomplished through respiratory, rather than laryngeal, means. (B) is incorrect because increased pitch range requires an increase in the tension of the vocal folds, which would not be accomplished by the chewing technique.

4. **(D)** The essential features of the facilitation process are scaffolding available repertoire and incorporation of new material into the total existing language system, so (D) is the correct answer. (A) is incorrect because the use of carrier phrases may be a helpful language intervention technique, but it does not necessarily build on the client's competence. (B) is incorrect

because behavior management may be a treatment technique, but it does not reflect the underlying theory addressed in this question. (C) is incorrect because prepackaged programs follow a set progression and, therefore, would not be facilitative. Facilitation enables self-learning from the available context, but prepackaged programs do not typically provide techniques addressing an individual client's unique pattern of language abilities.

5. **(C)** is the correct answer because it states the fundamental reason that standardized or normative instruments are useful in assessing a client's language and speech function. A client's behavior is most usefully compared to what is normal for a person in the same age range. (A) is incorrect because one might test a person before treatment and retest after treatment, but normative instruments do not chart precise increments of change for individual subjects. (B) is incorrect because developing specific objectives for therapeutic intervention is done after function has been assessed, and normative instruments typically do not provide the detailed information needed to develop specific objectives. (D) is incorrect because standardized instruments are not normally used to develop a description of client and milieu dimensions.

6. **(C)** Flaccid dysarthria and dysphagia are both disorders likely to be characterized by flaccidity or weakness of the oromotor and laryngeal mechanisms resulting from cranial nerve damage. These two disorders frequently coexist, so (C) is the correct answer. (A) is incorrect because aphasia is a language impairment that commonly results from cerebrovascular accidents. Although the neuromotor areas of the brain may also be affected by stroke, aphasia and dysphagia occur together relatively infrequently. Ataxic dysarthria is a neuromotor inability to coordinate motor activities. Swallowing requires coordination of muscular movement; however, dysphagia does not typically occur with the cerebellar damage associated with ataxia, so (B) is incorrect. (D) is incorrect because psychogenic mutism is not typically caused by a neurological disorder.

7. **(A)** The statement (A) is a reasonable standard to apply when judging whether a client has achieved generalization of a targeted skill. It shows that the client is exhibiting the skill independently in situations not covered during training, so (A) is the correct answer. (B) states that the client no longer needs cuing, so evidence of client progress is provided. A client might produce the targeted skill without cuing; however, the client still may be unable to produce it outside restricted clinical settings, so (B) is incorrect. (C) and (D) are incorrect because the client is in the process of learning and is still in need of cues and reinforcement.

8. **(A)** The most serious shortcoming of imitation as an intervention strategy is that imitation is not an intentionally communicative act, so (A) is the correct answer. (B) is incorrect because imitation does not necessarily rely on semantic knowledge. It is possible to imitate sequences of sounds without knowing what they mean. Imitation is controlled by the clinician, but that is not the most serious limitation of using imitation as an intervention strategy.

Therefore (C) is incorrect. (D) is incorrect because imitated speech is not necessarily contextualized.

9. **(B)** Naturalistic teaching focuses on the successful production of utterances that are communicatively useful in context, so (B) is the correct answer. Such utterances do not need to be syntactically complex, adult initiated, or child initiated, so (A) and (D) are incorrect. Multiple trials and training techniques are structured, not naturalistic, activities, so (C) is incorrect.

10. **(D)** Children with a history of prelingual otitis media are at risk for a mild to moderate conductive hearing loss and its effects on phonological production. Individuals with hearing loss often have difficulty perceiving strident or high-frequency consonants, such as sibilants. In speech they also typically fail to produce these consonants, since they do not perceive them, so (D) is the correct answer. (A) and (B) are incorrect because velar and glide deviation are not necessarily related to hearing loss. Nasal deviation is not a feature of the speech of children with a history of otitis media, so (C) is incorrect.

11. **(C)** Children with language disorders tend to ask fewer open-ended questions than do children who are developing normally, so (C) is the correct answer. The other answer choices, (A), (B), and (D), identify aspects of discourse that are characteristic of children who are developing normally or are the opposite of patterns seen in children with language disorders.

12. **(C)** There are empirical data that demonstrate that thermal stimulation

results in temporary facilitation of the swallowing reflex, so (C) is the correct answer. Cricopharyngeal myotomy serves to open the upper esophageal sphincter but does not facilitate the swallowing reflex, so (A) is incorrect. The chin tuck (B), and the Mendelsson maneuver, a technique for elevating the larynx (D), do not decrease delayed swallowing reflexes, so these answer choices are incorrect.

13. **(D)** The most important and most basic treatment goal for a client with a laryngectomy is restoration of oral communication, no matter how it is addressed, so (D) is the correct answer. Although the other answer choices, (A), (B), and (C), are viable options, each choice depends on the particular situation or patient. Only the broader goal of restoration of communication applies to all situations.

14. **(D)** The boy's deficits as noted are most indicative of a neurological disorder, and a neurologist could best provide the additional diagnostic information needed. Therefore (D) is the correct answer. The boy could have additional psychological or emotional problems, but those would be secondary issues, so (A) is incorrect. (B) is incorrect because the range of the child's difficulties is beyond the specialized knowledge of an otolaryngologist. There is no indication that a physical therapist would be in a position to provide appropriate diagnostic advice, so (C) is incorrect.

15. **(A)** Children with specific language impairments typically have difficulty producing utterances that are morphologically and syntactically well formed, so (A) is the correct answer. Children with specific language impairments also

have little trouble with the comprehension of phrases and short sentences, so (C) is incorrect. In addition, they display little trouble with the motor aspects of writing, so (D) is incorrect. (B) is incorrect because acquisition of basic word meanings is less likely to be impaired than inflectional morphology and syntax.

16. **(D)** The wording of (D) represents a well-written diagnostic statement for a child with communication problems that are physiological in nature. All of the other answer choices fail to demonstrate the presence of a physiological problem, so (D) is the correct answer. (A) is incorrect because mentioning the fact that the child's dentition is within normal limits would not satisfy the requirements of the requested diagnostic statement and, indeed, would suggest normal physical aspects of functioning. (B) is incorrect because that statement identifies a delay but not the physiological reason. (C) is incorrect because it gives no evidence to conclude that the child has a disorder.

17. **(D)** The statement in (D) appropriately focuses on a real-life situation concerning the use of the telephone and also defines a target percentage of trials; this will allow the clinician to determine whether the objective has been successfully met. Therefore (D) is the correct answer. (A) is incorrect because naming pictures does not define a functional activity in an applied context. (B) is incorrect because no level of successful behavior to be attained has been set and because the objective is not linked to functional communication behavior. Although the reduction of literal paraphasias might

be functional in improving successful communication of messages, this is not stated clearly. Therefore (C) is incorrect.

18. **(D)** Cerebrovascular accidents are statistically the leading cause of neurological speech and language disorders in the general adult population, so (D) is the correct answer. The events listed in the other answer choices of (A), (B), and (C) are less-frequent causes of neurological disorders.

19. **(D)** The specification outlined in (D) is included in the ASHA Code of Ethics. The details noted in the other answer choices, (A), (B), and (C), although they might be reasonable depending on the circumstances, are not specifically required by the Code of Ethics.

20. **(D)** The child as described is showing normal development except for problems in localizing environmental sounds. This symptom is indicative of a possible auditory problem, making it appropriate for the child to be referred to an audiologist for evaluation of auditory function, so (D) is the correct answer. (A) is incorrect because the case history gives no indication of psychological problems and the child is only 9 months old. (B) and (C) are incorrect because there is no diagnosed hearing loss.

21. **(D)** It would be most efficient for the speech-language pathologist to define the phonological processes in operation and address them through minimal-contrast pairs, so (D) is the correct answer. (A) is incorrect because the process is inefficient. (B) is incorrect because there may be no relationship

between the sounds the child can make and those the child cannot make. (C) is incorrect because auditory discrimination is not a sufficient strategy to correct the errors.

22. **(C)** By the nature of their conditions, children with brain injuries typically have greater difficulty managing their deficits than do children with learning disabilities, so (C) is the correct answer. The other answer choices are statements that do not accurately or reliably compare the disabilities of the two groups. Typically, both disabilities equally produce difficulties in social skills and information overload, so (B) and (D) are incorrect. (A) is incorrect because the amount of teaching and cueing depends more on the severity of the disorder and on individual factors such as motivation, and thus is not a differentiating factor between disorder etiologies.

23. **(A)** If an individual is responding randomly on a two-choice task, then there should be no significant preponderance of correct responses over incorrect responses. A result of 51% represents such an expected pattern of random responses, so (A) is the correct answer. (B) and (C) are incorrect because these outcomes would be characterized by significantly larger rates of correct responses. (D) is incorrect because there is no reason to believe that readiness to progress to a three-picture pointing task has been demonstrated.

24. **(A)** Stroboscopy is generally the most efficient and effective instrumentation for viewing the vocal folds during phonation, so (A) is the correct answer. Endoscopy could give a view of the

vocal folds during phonation, but stroboscopy provides a more detailed picture, so (B) is incorrect. (C) and (D) are incorrect because x-rays will not display the vibratory patterns of the vocal folds.

25. **(A)** A clinician who employs active listening responds to both the content and the affect (the emotional effect) of a client's remarks, so (A) is the correct answer. (B) is incorrect because note taking would interfere with engagement and it would not be active. In a clinician-directed interview, the clinician would be leading the discussion, and thus not in a position to engage in effective active listening, thus (C) is incorrect. (D) is incorrect because directing the client to specific answers is antithetical to listening, as this would seriously interfere with the client's spontaneous communication.

26. **(C)** The regulations governing the administration of Medicare for such a patient specify an assessment and a treatment. This treatment plan must be signed by the patient's physician every 9 weeks as long as treatment is necessary, so (C) is the correct response. The provisions listed in the other answer choices, (A), (B), and (D), are not required in this case and are not used as a basis for reimbursement.

27. **(A)** Using chronological ages as a performance criterion for a child with Down syndrome would make the child's language disorders seem more pronounced, so (A) is the correct answer and (B) is incorrect. (C) and (D) are incorrect because mental age is neither an error-free measurement nor a consistent correlate of verbal performance.

28. **(A)** By definition, athetosis is a type of cerebral palsy characterized by slow, arrhythmic, writhing, and involuntary movements of the extremities, so (A) is the correct answer. Spasticity involves jerky, uncontrolled movements with increased muscular tone, so (B) is incorrect. Hypotonia involves muscular weakness, but not the other symptoms listed, so (C) is incorrect. Rigidity involves a functional lack of movement, so (D) is incorrect.

29. **(C)** In apraxia of speech, the appropriate coordination of motor movements required to produce well-formed speech sounds is impaired. Clients with apraxia generally have adequate language comprehension, muscular power, and general body coordination. Treatment for this condition appropriately emphasizes auditory-visual stimulation, oral-motor repetition, and phonetic placement, so (C) is the correct answer. (A) is incorrect because apraxia neither results in impairment of respiration or difficulty with phonation. Apraxia does not lead to deficits in comprehension or problems with pitch or vocal intensity, so (B) and (D) are incorrect.

30. **(B)** For an individual diagnosed with a moderate fluency disorder, recent graduation from college and preparation to seek employment constitute evidence of a considerable degree of self-motivation. This implies a favorable prognosis for treatment, so (B) is the correct answer. (A) is incorrect because the client's activities more than a decade earlier would be relatively unimportant when considering the client's current prognosis. The tension created by an employer's request that the client improve might make the

fluency disorder even worse, so (C) is incorrect. (D) is incorrect because a client's self-appraisal could make the client more likely to resent the treatment regimen.

31. **(B)** HIPAA stipulates limitations on sharing of patient medical information between health insurance agencies, therefore (B) is the correct answer. The actions in (A), (C), and (D) are permitted under HIPAA, so these answers are incorrect.

32. **(C)** An independent variable is manipulated or varied by the investigator to measure its effect on the dependent variable(s). Watson and Hughes manipulated vocal loudness to determine its effect on prosodic F_0 and durational variables. Therefore, (C) is the correct answer. (A) and (D) are incorrect since those variables were not part of the Watson and Hughes study. (B) is incorrect, as both F_0 declination and final-word lengthening represent dependent variables that were measured as an outcome of vocal variations in loudness.

33. **(C)** In the conclusion of the abstract, Watson and Hughes suggest a relationship between increased vocal loudness and improvement in communicative effectiveness in some persons with dysarthria. This relationship is not directly supported by their study, as individuals with dysarthria were not tested, so (C) is the correct answer. (A) and (B) are incorrect as they do not address the relationship of dysarthria, vocal loudness, and improved communicative effectiveness. (D) is incorrect for the same reason and, furthermore, the results were found to be statistically significant.

34. **(D)** Watson and Hughes use the same group of participants who recite a paragraph under three conditions: "normal," "twice-normal," and "half-normal" loudness. This is an example of a within-subjects design, in which the dependent variables (in this case, prosodic F_0 and durational variables) are measured repeatedly in the same participants under different task conditions (in this case, vocal loudness). Therefore, (D) is the correct answer. (A) is incorrect because a longitudinal design would require tracking change in the dependent variables over time. (B) is incorrect, as the study included no baseline measures. (C) is incorrect because there was one single group of participants.

35. **(D)** A 4-year-old child should have already developed final consonants, and there is no reason to expect that final consonants would emerge during the following year without intervention. (D) is therefore the correct answer, and (A) is incorrect. Treatment for /p/ would address only one phoneme, and a phonological approach is more productive than single-sound remediation. Also, there is no indication that the child has particular difficulty producing plosives. (B), therefore, is incorrect. There is no indication of cognitive dysfunction, since the child simply has a phonological processing disorder with significant delay, so (C) is incorrect.

36. **(A)** The client has a resonance and phonation disorder indicative of velopharyngeal and laryngeal problems. The velopharyngeal problem could be assisted by prosthetic or surgical intervention, so (A) is the correct answer. (B) is incorrect because strengthening exercises for the oral articulators are not effective for improving velopharyngeal function. Neither the yawn-sigh technique (a relaxation technique) or vocal rest is appropriate when vocal fold adduction is weak, so (C) and (D) are incorrect.

37. **(A)** When the task is to reinforce a behavior that has already been acquired, a random ratio of tokens to correct responses creates an intermittent reinforcement schedule and is the most effective. Such a reinforcement schedule would decrease the client's dependence on the token reward, so (A) is the correct answer. A ratio of one token to one response is effective for the acquisition of new behaviors, but not for reinforcement of learned behaviors, so (B) is incorrect. (C) also maintains dependence on the token reinforcement, and (D) maintains the expectation that a reward will regularly be given, so those answer choices are incorrect.

38. **(C)** Construction of a palatal lift appliance is appropriate for a patient with flaccid paralysis characterized by an intact palate that does not function, so (C) is the correct answer. When a submucous cleft palate creates a speech problem, the first choice of treatment would be surgical, so (A) is incorrect. Surgery would be the first choice for treatment for an unrepaired cleft of the secondary palate or a congenitally short palate, so (B) and (D) are incorrect.

39. **(D)** For an infant with moderate sensorineural hearing loss, parents are in the best position to provide consistent auditory stimulation, and such stimulation is what the infant needs to develop awareness of sound. Therefore

(D) is the correct answer. Infants are at the prelinguistic developmental level would not be developing articulation skills, and there is no reason to suspect cognitive problems, so (A) and (B) are incorrect. The parent-infant relationship is the primary social interaction, so it would be too early to focus on the development of social skills, thus (C) is incorrect.

40. **(C)** The child has a behavioral problem that should be evaluated for the purpose of identification and management planning, so (C) is the correct answer. Simply rejecting the referral to the speech-language pathologist would not ensure appropriate treatment and evaluation for the child, so (A) is incorrect. It is possible that the child has undiagnosed problems that are contributing to the behavior, so addressing the behavior itself as in (B), might not be adequate. (D) is incorrect because, although there appears to be pragmatic language problems, there is no other evidence for a primary speech or language disorder. Because the child is exhibiting problems that may involve other factors, team evaluation and consideration of the results would be necessary before any type of treatment is initiated.

41. **(D)** Naturalistic contexts or everyday situations provide opportunities for the use of functional and meaningful linguistic forms, so (D) is the correct answer. The other answer choices represent tasks or approaches that can be used in language intervention but do not promote use of the linguistic forms in everyday life situations as efficiently and effectively as intervention embedded in naturalistic contexts. Thus (A), (B), and (C) are incorrect.

42. **(B)** is the correct answer because it expresses an accurate distinction between the terms *agent* and *subject* as they are used to describe language. (A) is incorrect because the agent does not necessarily agree with the verb. For example, in the sentence, "The dogs were tickled by the boy," the subject is "the dogs" and the agent is "the boy." However, the verb agrees with the plurality of the subject (*dogs*), not with the singularity of the agent (*boy*). (C) is incorrect because it inaccurately suggests that the agent of an utterance cannot always be determined. By definition, a sentence must have at least an implied subject, so (D) is incorrect.

43. **(C)** Eustachian tube dysfunction, a major factor contributing to middle-ear disease and conductive hearing loss, is nearly universal in infants with cleft palates, so (C) is the correct answer. Inability to create positive pressure in the oral cavity describes problems in sucking, not hearing, so (A) is incorrect. It is usually Eustachian tube dysfunction rather than malformation of the middle ear ossicles or cochlear dysfunction that contributes to the hearing problems of infants with cleft palate, so (B) and (D) are incorrect.

44. **(D)** Treatment in consultation with the patient's primary-care physician or medical team would provide the information needed to determine the best management of the patient, so (D) is the correct answer. Treatment on a monthly basis may or may not be adequate, and there is no reason to believe that monthly treatment would be effective, so (A) is incorrect. The patient's physician would not necessarily know what speech-language treatment is required, so (B) is incor-

rect. (C) is incorrect because there is no need to avoid physical contact with the patient as long as universal precautions are followed.

45. **(A)** The treatment goal expressed in (A), the correct answer choice, represents a real-life, naturalistic use of communication skills. Since pragmatics is the study of language in such realistic contexts, (B) is incorrect because it would involve an attempt by the clinician to increase the mean length of utterance in a nonfunctional context not related to pragmatics. (C) represents a goal related to incorporating a learned articulation pattern into conversation, but this is also not a skill related directly to pragmatics, so (C) is incorrect. Telling a story does represent a pragmatic situation; however, the goal connected to this situation is morphological not pragmatic, so (D) is incorrect.

46. **(D)** This client's language reflects anomia. Treatment to remediate these difficulties is appropriate, so (D) is the correct answer. The client has already experienced at least 3 months of spontaneous recovery, and treatment should not be delayed until further spontaneous recovery has occurred. In fact, treatment during the period of spontaneous recovery is highly recommended, so (A) is incorrect. The problem will not be addressed by having the client communicate in writing rather than speaking, so (B) is incorrect. The client's dysfluency is apparently due to his word-retrieval problem and is expected to be resolved from treatment of the problem, so (C) is incorrect.

47. **(A)** Sufficient hydration for this patient will be accomplished by a PEG tube

only, so (A) is the correct answer. The other answer choices, (B), (C), and (D), offer an amount of hydration in meager amounts that would be insufficient for this patient regardless of the thickness or thinness of the liquids.

48. **(B)** Early language stimulation is best provided by the infant's primary caregivers, and those individuals require direction to promote the infant's learning. (B) is therefore the correct answer. The activities listed in the other answer choices, (A), (C), and (D), are all more appropriate for later developmental stages.

49. **(B)** An assessment of the problem must be undertaken before treatment is provided, and the best way to do this is to obtain a modified barium-swallow study. Therefore (B) is the correct answer. All of the other answer choices, (A), (C), and (D), represent actions that might be taken after the results of the assessment have been determined. Proceeding with any of these treatment options before the appropriate study has been completed could be dangerous to the patient's health.

50. **(A)** The child needs to be encouraged to proceed to the two-word production stage, and the use of pretend play will encourage action/object two-word phrases such as "Feed baby" and "Brush hair." (A) is therefore the correct answer. The other answer choices, (B), (C), and (D), involve behaviors that do not necessarily promote language behaviors.

51. **(D)** Ms. Lopez' phonological errors are due to voicing, which is not a presumed effect of foreign accent, so (D) is the correct answer. Within each

pair, the error sound and the correct sound are identical in manner, place, and frication, so (A), (B), and (C) are incorrect.

52. **(D)** Ms. Helene has a suspected neurological disorder and she achieves a score that is below the norms for individuals her age. Given this information alone, the most that can be said is that she has difficulty with naming. The precise nature of her deficit cannot be determined, so (D) is the correct answer. The other answer choices, (A), (B), and (C), make unsubstantiated assumptions about the patient's disorder.

53. **(A)** A single exposure of several hours to continuous music above 100 dB SPL will most likely produce tinnitus and a temporary threshold shift in the high frequencies, so (A) is the correct answer. A temporary threshold shift will not affect speech perception, so (B) is incorrect. A temporary threshold shift occurs in the higher frequencies, so (C) is incorrect. A single exposure at this level would be insufficient to result in a permanent threshold shift, so (D) is incorrect.

54. **(B)** Given the language sample, the child incorrectly regularizes the past tense forms of irregular verbs, so (B) is the correct answer. (A) and (C) are incorrect because the child has provided evidence of using adjectives and prepositional phrases correctly. Conjunctions and embedding are above the child's developmental level; therefore, (D) is incorrect.

55. **(D)** Mr. Charles has Alzheimer's disease with memory loss and deteriorating language skills. Treatment should be designed to help his caregivers improve

the conditions related to his basic communication needs in his immediate environment. Speech and language treatment alone is very unlikely to be effective and thus is not appropriate, so (D) is the correct answer and (A), (B), and (C) are incorrect.

56. **(A)** Since the principal is provided with a justification detailing the needs of the students' treatment and the plan does not leave students without services, (A) is the correct answer. It is inappropriate to refer students to a private practitioner because the parents would be required to pay for therapy, so (B) is incorrect. Suggesting a speech-language pathologist from another school district would be inappropriate, so (C) is incorrect. There was space for an additional student on the caseload, so there is no reason to maintain the current caseload of 34, so (D) is incorrect.

57. **(A)** The objective listed in (A) refers to speech sounds in general distinctive-feature classes, rather than in isolated phonemes or overly specific classifications, so this is the correct answer. (B) is incorrect because it focuses on the production of only one class of sounds. (C) is incorrect because it focuses on a developmental approach. (D) is incorrect because it focuses on a single sound.

58. **(D)** The morphological feature listed in (D) is an acceptable utterance in African-American English (AAE) but not Standard American English (SAE), which, if scored as incorrect, would pose an unfair penalty on the speaker of AAE, so (D) is the correct answer. The features listed in (A), (B), and (C) would be inappropriate for both AAE and SAE, thus indicating grammatical errors rather than a dialectal difference.

59. **(D)** The client has an advanced stage of amyotrophic lateral sclerosis, which results in progressive deterioration of communication abilities. An augmentative communication system is now, and will continue to be, the best option for improving or maintaining communication for this client, so (D) is the correct answer. Although the treatments in (A), (B), and (C) may be helpful for clients with one or more of the problems, if they occurred in isolation for a client with deteriorating communication skills, such treatments would be of temporary value, if any.

60. **(B)** The cognitive skills of a child at the one-word stage will most strongly influence the child's speech-language responses, so language intervention for the child should take into account the child's cognitive skills, and (B) is the correct answer. Motor skills would affect articulation rather than language so (A) is incorrect. Syntactic skills are irrelevant at this stage, since syntax is not displayed during the one-word stage. Therefore (C) is incorrect. Language skills can develop despite serious articulation problems, so (D) is incorrect.

61. **(C)** Computer software and other aids are not meant to replace treatment sessions provided by a speech-language pathologist but rather to enhance clients' opportunities to improve their skills in relation to goals established by the clinician; thus, (C) is the correct answer. (A), (B), and (D) all suggest that the computer software would in some way replace direct contact with the speech-language pathologist and are incorrect.

62. **(A)** The symptoms listed are indicative of deficits that are generally associated with right-hemisphere dysfunction, so (A) is the correct answer. A left-hemisphere cerebrovascular accident might produce these symptoms in some left-handed individuals, but rarely, so (B) is incorrect. The symptoms indicate a problem in only one hemisphere. Since (C) and (D) involve both hemispheres, they are incorrect.

63. **(D)** It would be appropriate to provide speech and language services with the objective of reducing and eliminating the speech production errors exhibited by the patient, so (D) is the correct answer. (A), (B), and (C) represent actions that are premature considering it has been 2 months since surgery occurred. Many patients benefit from speech treatment services immediately following surgery.

64. **(D)** Information about the development of older siblings, while sometimes useful, does not provide the objective, documented evidence required to justify provision of treatment so (D) is the correct answer. (A), (B), and (C) are incorrect because they involve information that the speech-language pathologist can observe directly and report regarding the child's disorder.

65. **(D)** The nature and frequency of the child's dysfluent behaviors will help distinguish normal nonfluency from stuttering, so (D) is the correct answer. The nature of the dysfluency includes such behaviors as anticipatory struggle and avoidance behaviors. The presence or absence of these features can help distinguish developmental nonfluent speech from true stuttering. (B) is incorrect because the amount of talking the child does during the assessment is not relevant as long as the child

produces a substantive speech sample. (A) and (C) are incorrect because the length of time the child has been dysfluent or the rate at which the child talks are less critical when making the differential diagnosis.

66. **(C)** A test that has interjudge reliability is one whose results are replicable, even if different people administer the test. Therefore (C) is the correct answer. (A) is incorrect because age norms establish developmental milestones related to the test's results. They in no way ensure that the results of the test will be replicable. (B) is incorrect because content validity establishes whether the test measures the skills it was intended to measure, not whether the test's results are replicable. (D) is incorrect because split-half reliability involves dividing a test into two equivalent halves. As speech and language tests usually measure developmental progress, the items are typically not amenable to being grouped into equivalent halves.

67. **(D)** A nursing home resident in a late stage of progressive dementia would most need assistance from the speech-language pathologist in helping caregivers assist the resident with daily communication functions, so (D) is the correct answer. (A), (B), and (C) list treatment goals that would be inappropriate for a person with a progressive disease at this stage.

68. **(C)** Of the muscles listed, the crico-thyroid muscle has the greatest control over the fundamental frequency of the laryngeal tone by lengthening and tensing the vocal folds, so (C) is the correct answer. The posterior cricoaryntenoid (A) abducts the vocal folds. The lateral cricoarytenoid (B)

adducts the vocal folds. The hyoglossus (D) lowers the tongue. Therefore (A), (B), and (D) are incorrect.

69. **(D)** Manual depression of the larynx will lengthen the vocal folds, causing them to vibrate at a lower frequency, so (D) is the correct answer. Development of phonation from coughing is a treatment that brings about adduction of the vocal folds and is appropriate for aphonia, so (A) is incorrect. Pushing exercises also promote adduction of the vocal folds, putting them in a state ready for phonation, but do not affect the frequency at which they vibrate, so (B) is incorrect. Auditory training will not significantly improve self-monitoring of laryngeal pitch for a client with severe bilateral hearing loss and, in any case would not have a direct effect on phonation, so (C) is incorrect.

70. **(D)** Speaking while alternately leaving the nostrils open and pinching them closed is an easy way for a speaker to determine whether inappropriate nasal airflow is occurring, so (D) is the correct answer. This technique allows one to determine the difference in airflow pattern when speech is produced with the nostrils occluded as compared with speech produced when the nostrils are open. For a speaker with velopharyngeal incompetence, closure of the nostrils will eliminate the nasal airflow in production of /s/. (A) is incorrect because looking in a mirror while speaking provides no useful information related to nasal airflow. Holding a feather in front of the mouth while speaking does allow a speaker to determine whether there is oral airflow, and this could be helpful, for example, in showing whether stops

are aspirated. However, this, technique is not useful for determining nasal airflow, so (B) is incorrect. Being aware of vowel-sound productions is not useful in determining airflow patterns, so (C) is incorrect.

71. **(D)** Psychological counseling is most appropriate for a client who appears interested in improving speech but has not been motivated long enough to complete the several treatment programs already begun. The client also does not exhibit maintenance of benefits from prior treatment. Thus, psychological counseling should precede any further remedial efforts, and (D) is the correct answer. There is nothing in the client's history to support continued efforts by the client or clinician without psychological intervention, so (A), (B), and (C) are incorrect.

72. **(D)** Gastrostomy involves the opening of a stoma in the stomach wall when normal food ingestion is impossible or ill advised. This procedure is of little value in assessing swallowing. Therefore, (D) is the correct answer. Videofluoroscopy is useful in assessing swallowing because it can identify the specific nature of oropharyngeal dysphagia. It can define abnormality of movements, trace the progress of the bolus, and demonstrate aspiration, so (A) is incorrect. (B) is incorrect because bedside evaluation, although it cannot directly assess swallowing, can help define oral abnormalities and pharyngeal wall impairments. (C) is incorrect because fiberoptic endoscopy is also useful in assessing swallowing by providing direct observation of pharyngeal activity during the swallowing process.

73. **(D)** According to mourning theory, a person in grief is most receptive to accepting new information about the source of grief when the person has just entered the recovery stage. Therefore (D) is the correct answer. (A) and (B) are incorrect because they represent a time period when the parents would still be experiencing shock and denial about their child's condition, and they could be unreceptive to detailed information concerning assessment and treatment plans. (C) is incorrect because it represents a stage of the mourning process during which the parents would still be experiencing emotional trauma, and thus would not be ready to process detailed information.

74. **(C)** Ear malformation is the only symptom among those listed that is typical of hemifacial microsomia, a genetic diagnosis within the oculo-auricular-vertebral (OAV) spectrum. Therefore (C) is the correct answer. None of the other conditions listed, (A), (B), and (D), are typical of this syndrome.

75. **(D)** Words containing combinations of phonemes similar to those into which the child makes the inappropriate insertion would be most helpful for this child, so (D) is the correct answer. (A) is incorrect because there is no indication that the words relating to the child's environment would have relevant relationships to the error sounds. (B) is incorrect because the error occurs in monosyllabic words, so syllabicity is not the appropriate environment. (C) is incorrect because the statement relating to the distinctive features of sounds is too broad to be useful.

76. **(D)** Since a conductive hearing loss can contribute to delayed expressive language development, (D) is the correct answer given Michael's history of recurrent middle-ear infections. An otolaryngologist would be able to clinically manage otitis media and make provisions to obtain an audiological assessment. (A) is incorrect because Michael's preschool and educational issues are not of immediate need. (B) is incorrect because there is no indication of neurologic disease. (C) is incorrect because the history does not suggest the presence of socioemotional disorder.

77. **(A)** Articulation characterized by struggle, inconsistency, and errors of sound and syllable sequencing strongly suggest developmental apraxia of speech, so the correct answer is (A). Although Michael has a history of recurring middle-ear infections, (B) is incorrect because a conductive hearing loss would typically result in consistent and predictable articulation errors. (C) is incorrect because dysarthria would be associated with both volitional and nonvolitional deficits, and none were observed during feeding. Age-appropriate receptive language skills and deficits in oral motor function are not consistent with specific language impairment, so (D) is incorrect.

78. **(D)** Michael's case history suggests his poor intelligibility is tied to his inconsistent sequencing of speech sounds and syllables. Therefore (D) is the most appropriate answer. (B) is incorrect because Michael's receptive language skills were found to be age appropriate. As spontaneous oral movements are apparently intact, gross motor support and muscle weakness are not an issue. Therefore (A) and (C) are incorrect.

79. **(A)** Toddlers and preschoolers respond better to games and play activities than to structured exercises, so (A) is the correct answer, and (C) is incorrect. (B) is incorrect because there is no indication that Michael's speech and language deficits would be addressed by self-monitoring and because children of Michael's age have limited meta-linguistic awareness. (D) is incorrect because continuing deficits support continued early-intervention services.

80. **(B)** Clients have the right to review their own records, so (B) is the correct answer. There are no restrictions that limit release of client records only to other health care professionals or only by subpoena, so (A) and (D) are incorrect. There are also no laws that allow the release of such sensitive personal records to anyone who submits a formal written request, so (C) is incorrect.

81. **(B)** Having the client use light and gentle vocal-fold contacts will help to reduce tension, and thus would be effective in treating hyperadduction of the vocal folds, so (B) is the correct answer. All of the other answer choices, (A), (C), and (D), are incorrect because the actions listed would serve to increase vocal tension.

82. **(B)** Consonant cluster reduction is the most persistent of the normal developmental processes listed, so (B) is the correct answer. (A), (B), and (C) are less likely to be persistent.

83. **(C)** Whispered speech is composed largely of aperiodic sounds, as the vocal folds do not vibrate while whispering is taking place. (C) is therefore the correct answer. Approximating the

arytenoid cartilages so that their medial surfaces are in direct contact would result in normal phonation, so (A) is incorrect. Aperiodic sounds by definition have no periodicity, and thus no specifiable fundamental frequency, so (B) is incorrect. Despite the fact that they have no fundamental frequency, whispered vowels do have discernible formants; the supralaryngeal vocal tract reinforces the amplitudes of whispered aperiodic vowels at virtually the same resonant frequency ranges as it does for the same vowels produced by laryngeal tone. Therefore (D) is incorrect.

84. **(B)** Syntactic complexity is determined by the number of transformational rules that are applied to a given sentence. "John is helping Bill" is a simple declarative sentence and has no transformations, so (D) is incorrect. Inverting the verb to form a question (A) and adding negation (C) constitute transformations. Thus, the sentence in each of these options has undergone one transformation. The sentence in (B) involves inversion, negation, and an interrogative word, so with three transformations, (B) has the greatest syntactic complexity and is the correct answer.

85. **(C)** The child is using compensatory glottal stops, mid-dorsum palatal stops, and pharyngeal fricatives. She has had surgical management to correct velopharyngeal incompetence. She now needs to produce the stops and fricatives for which she is making compensations. Therefore, articulation treatment is appropriate, and (C) is the correct answer. Determining the cause of the persistent articulation errors is the responsibility of the speech-language pathologist, not

the entire cleft palate team, so (A) is incorrect. Speech treatment should precede any consideration for revision of a pharyngeal flap, so (B) is incorrect. Teaching a soft glottal attack would be used in voice treatment for a person who has hoarse voice quality due to vocal nodules. This child, however, is producing compensatory glottal stops, so such an intervention would be ineffective, so (D) is incorrect.

86. **(D)** According to developmental norms, /k/ is the target phoneme that should be selected for intervention, so (D) is the correct answer. All of the other phonemes listed appear later in the developmental sequence. Therefore (A), (B), and (C) are incorrect.

87. **(B)** Impaired attention and memory are consistent with the brain injury sustained by the client, so (B) is the correct answer. There is no evidence for any of the other areas of potential deficit listed in the other answer choices. Therefore, (A), (C), and (D) are incorrect.

88. **(B)** The child is exhibiting symptoms indicative of Williams syndrome, so (B) is the correct answer. (A) is incorrect because the child is described as sociable (suggesting adequate self-concept), and his appearance, although distinctive in certain traits as described, is still normal. The child is not exhibiting symptoms of a chromosomal abnormality, nor Marshall syndrome, so (C) and (D) are incorrect.

89. **(B)** Changing beliefs about self-control and the perceived benefits of stuttering represent the only answer choice that is cognitive in nature, so (B) is the correct answer. The other answer choices,

(A), (C), and (D), focus on behavioral conditioning or other client characteristics that are not cognitive in nature.

90. **(B)** A multimodal approach offers more communicative options than any of the other approaches listed, so (B) is the correct answer. A unimodal and bimodal approach offer fewer options; therefore, (A) and (C) are incorrect. (D) is incorrect because a vocal system is not a consideration for vocabulary, seating, positioning and control.

91. **(D)** Melodic intonation therapy (MIT) is a procedure appropriately used by speech-language pathologists to promote specific results. The speech-language pathologist has responsibility for determining the value of this procedure in relation to the objectives of the speech and language treatment program, so (D) is the correct answer. It would be unreasonable either to provide or to refuse to provide MIT on the basis of the physician's recommendation without considering the appropriateness of the procedure for the patient, so (A) and (B) are incorrect. Although a physician is not normally in a position to prescribe speech-language services, there is no need for the speech-language pathologist to take the confrontational approach toward the physician in (C), so that answer choice is incorrect.

92. **(A)** Wernicke's aphasia results in deficits related to the ability to recognize the adequacy of one's verbal production, so (A) is the correct answer. Singing as an aphasia treatment approach is not suitable for people with the posterior lesions associated with Wernicke's aphasia, so (B) is incorrect. Wernicke's aphasia does not render an

individual nonverbal, and the verbal output associated with it often includes syntactically complex sentence structures, so (C) and (D) are incorrect.

93. **(D)** The symptoms exhibited by this client represent a classic profile of a person who has contact ulcers, so (D) is the correct answer. The identifying characteristics are the personality of the individual and the presence of glottal fry. Glottal fry is not a characteristic of any of the other answer choices. With acute laryngitis, a person may lose the use of the voice and may even become aphonic during the episode of laryngitis, but does not exhibit glottal fry, so (C) is incorrect. With ventricular phonation, a person is using the false vocal folds, a rough type of phonation that, when used in conjunction with the true vocal folds, can result in diplophonia, but the symptoms do not include glottal fry, so (B) is incorrect. Spastic dysphonia involves aphonic breaks due to sudden overadduction or underadduction of the vocal folds, but no glottal fry, so (A) is incorrect.

94. **(A)** Overshooting or undershooting of an intended target is typical of individuals with deficits related to a lesion of the cerebellum, so (A) is the correct answer. The symptoms listed in (B), (C), and (D) are indeed characteristic of brain damage but are not specifically indicative of a lesion of the cerebellum, so those answer choices are incorrect.

95. **(A)** Development of phonation through coughing or throat clearing is an effective technique in the treatment of aphonia, so (A) is the correct answer. Aphonia is cause by abduction of the vocal folds, so patients should be encouraged to adduct the vocal folds

by coughing or throat clearing and then to produce phonation. Clients with aphonia are usually convinced that they cannot produce phonation, so asking them to develop a hard glottal attack, to alternate voiceless and voiced sibilants, or to try easy initiation of phonation would be unlikely to result in phonation. Therefore, (B), (C), and (D) are incorrect.

96. **(B)** Developmental norms derive from the percentage of children at a given age who correctly articulate sounds, so (B) is correct. Developmental norms provide no information about reading skills, frequency of occurrence of the sound, or learning ability, so (A), (C), and (D) are incorrect.

97. **(D)** Linguistic performance typically lags behind linguistic competence, so (D) is the correct answer, and (C) is incorrect. The child in this case is competent to perceive the difference between the phonemes /r/ and /w/ when spoken by others but not capable of producing the sound. (A) and (B) are incorrect because the child demonstrates ability to comprehend the semantic differences.

98. **(A)** A child with developmental apraxia would not have difficulties with chewing, eating, and swallowing, whereas a child with flaccid dysarthria is likely to have such difficulties, so (A) is the correct answer. The characteristics listed in (B), (C), and (D) could occur in either disorder but would not serve to differentiate the disorders, so those answer choices are all incorrect.

99. **(C)** Genetic factors interacting with environmental influences represents the etiology of cleft palate, so (C) is

the correct answer, and (A) and (B) are incorrect. The mother's consumption of alcohol during pregnancy is a possible etiology of cleft palate, but it is an example of an environmental influence that does not, in itself, explain the full etiology of cleft palate, so (D) is incorrect.

100. **(B)** There are two ways to interpret the structure of the sentence "Visiting friends can be a nuisance." One interpretation is that it is bothersome to visit friends. The other is that friends who have come for a visit are bothersome. This sentence, therefore, would be appropriate as part of a test of a person's ability to recognize syntactic ambiguity, and (B) is the correct answer. The sample sentence is complete, not a fragment, so (A) is incorrect. The sentence does not contain metaphorical usages, so (C) is incorrect. The sentence also does not contain any common homonyms, so (D) is incorrect.

101. **(B)** Prostheses such as those developed by Blom-Singer and Panje shunt air from the trachea to the esophagus, allowing the air to be used in normal esophageal speech, so (B) is the correct answer. The prostheses do not produce the results listed in (A), (C), and (D), so those answer choices are incorrect.

102. **(D)** Anoxic encephalopathy is brain damage resulting from oxygen deprivation, which typically leads to a global impairment that affects memory. Memory deficits will affect all areas of communication and become the most significant. So, (D) is the correct answer. (A) and (C) are incorrect because they specify impairments that result from more-specific damage to

the brain. (B) is incorrect because dysphagia may be long term, but multiple compensatory management strategies are available.

103. **(D)** The primary consideration must be whether the client's stuttering was present before the CVA occurred. Dysfluent speech may or may not be directly related to the client's CVA, so (D) is the correct answer. (B) and (C) are secondary issues that may accompany either stuttering or the CVA, so those answer choices are incorrect. The site and extent of the lesion may help explain the stuttering only if it has been caused by the CVA, so (A) is incorrect.

104. **(C)** Conclusions from research reports are restricted to the variables examined in those studies. A relationship between poor auditory memory and language impairment has been found in some research investigations. Other factors could be involved, however, suggesting that further research is needed. Conclusions about treatment or the effects of the impairment must be made through additional research studies, so (C) is the correct answer. The research reports showed a relationship and did not examine intervention, so (A) is incorrect. These reports also did not examine the effects of treatment, so a conclusion about lack of improvement after treatment cannot be drawn, and (B) is incorrect. (D) is incorrect because it prescribes an evaluation and is not a conclusion that can be drawn from the studies.

105. **(C)** The primary goal of any intervention is to effectuate the best functional outcome for the client. Generalization with respect to the environments in

which the augmentative device is used effectively would help accomplish this goal, so (C) is the correct answer. Improving technical skills, as in (A) and (D), and hardware maintenance, as in (B), could be reasonable secondary goals but not primary goals, so those answer choices are incorrect.

106. **(D)** Perturbation is a disturbance of quality of the laryngeal tone, or fundamental frequency of the voice. When the cycle-to-cycle period changes abruptly, the laryngeal tone is distorted. A hoarse voice would be an example of such a perturbation. Therefore (D) is the correct answer. (A), (B), and (C) are incorrect because they refer to formant frequencies, not to the fundamental frequency.

107. **(C)** The valleculae are depressions that lie lateral to the median epiglottal folds. Pooling of liquids in the valleculae gives a person the feeling that there is material in the respiratory pathway, so coughing would be a natural reaction, and (C) is the correct answer. Nerve pain, or neuralgia, is rarely associated with dysphagia, so (D) is incorrect. The other answer choices are incorrect because they address symptoms related to dysphagia that are not a direct result of pooling of liquids in the valleculae.

108. **(A)** In normal development, a child begins to use vocalizations to express specific intentions at 10 months of age, so (A) is the correct answer. If an infant is developing typically, then reaching for objects, as in (B), and establishing joint reference, as in (C), will be accomplished at around 3 months. Therefore (C) and (D) are incorrect.

The use of recognizable words and phrases to express intention does not develop until after a child has established vocalization patterns, so (D) is incorrect.

109. **(B)** An ABAB single-case design allows the comparison of baseline performance to treatment outcomes, so (B) is the correct answer. Standardized assessment tools reveal how well a client performs compared to a specified population but do not provide direct information about the client's progress, so (A) is incorrect. A subjective-objective assessment plan (SOAP) explains a desired goal and specific outcomes in a given treatment session but does not measure the overall effects of intervention, so (C) is incorrect. Specific pretests examine criteria before intervention but yield no information about efficacy of treatment, so (D) is incorrect.

110. **(D)** Primary innervation to the larynx and velum is provided by the Xth cranial nerve, the vagus nerve, so (D) is the correct answer. The other answer choices identify cranial nerves that are not primarily involved in motor innervation to the larynx and velum. The Vth cranial nerve innervates the tensor veli palatini muscle. Therefore (A) is incorrect. The VIIth cranial nerve innervates muscles of the face, so (B) is incorrect. The IXth cranial nerve has some involvement in swallowing but does not supply the larynx or the velum, so (C) is incorrect.

111. **(D)** Auditory training focuses on the interpretation of auditory input and teaches a client to discriminate among speech sounds, so (D) is the correct

answer. The other answer choices, (A), (B), and (C) are incorrect because they include intervention involving the movements speech production. Such intervention would address output and would not be a main objective of an auditory training program.

112. **(D)** A child who has had repeated episodes of middle-ear infection is likely to have experienced periods of temporary hearing loss that can affect all domains of language acquisition, so (D) is the correct answer. (A), (B), and (C) are incorrect because they are each limited to one specific domain of language development.

113. **(C)** The midsagittal section shows that the speaker's velopharyngeal port is open, allowing a flow of air into the nasal cavity. The resulting lack of intraoral air pressure would not sustain normal production of the phoneme. Therefore (C) is the correct answer. The position of the incisors, as shown, is sufficiently appropriate for the production of the /f/, so (A) and (B) are incorrect. Likewise, lip placement for production of this phoneme is adequate as shown in the diagram, so (D) is incorrect.

114. **(C)** Medialization thyroplasty moves the paralyzed vocal fold closer to the midglottis to allow better compensation by the unaffected fold. Of the choices provided, only the production of a hard glottal attack addresses this compensatory behavior, so (C) is the correct answer. (A) and (B) are incorrect because these techniques are used to treat vocal hyperfunction, which is not the case for unilateral vocal fold paralysis. (D) is incorrect because

improved glottal competence is associated with decreasing airflow.

115. **(D)** Functional independence is a main goal for a client shortly before dismissal from treatment. This goal can be achieved by teaching compensatory strategies to minimize remaining deficits, so (D) is the correct answer. The other answer choices, (A), (B), and (C), are incorrect because they suggest deficit-specific treatments that would not lead directly to improvement in functional independence.

116. **(D)** Brown's morphemes are acquired by all children in a sequence that is determined by their semantic and syntactic complexity from simplest forms to the most complex forms, so (D) is the correct answer. Frequency of occurrence in adult speech does not affect acquisitional order, so (A) is incorrect. Ease of production is a consideration for the acquisition of phonemes, but children often acquire and use morphemes, even though they might not pronounce them correctly, so (B) is incorrect. (C) is incorrect because the use of figurative language is a pragmatic ability unrelated to the acquisition of Brown's morphemes.

117. **(B)** The director of a new speech and hearing clinic would most appropriately prospect for referrals by identifying major consumer groups and creating a plan to contact them, so (B) is the correct answer. It would be a violation of patient confidentiality for a hospital to provide the names of patients, so (A) is incorrect. It is a violation of the ASHA Code of Ethics to malign fellow professionals, so (C) is incorrect. The Code of Ethics does not prohibit the appropriate marketing of

speech and language services; however, passively waiting for demand to increase on its own is an ineffective and potentially ruinous business practice, so (D) is incorrect.

118. **(A)** The phoneme /ʃ/ is not within the phonemic inventory of the Spanish language. Hence, native speakers of Spanish typically substitute the affricate /tʃ/ when producing English words containing that phoneme. It can be assumed that a native speaker of Spanish would have made such a substitution before acquiring an anomic aphasia, so (A) is the correct answer. (B) and (C) are incorrect because the interference is phonological, not semantic. The client is identified as having an anomic aphasia, and phonemic paraphasias do not typically occur with that type of aphasia, so (D) is incorrect.

119. **(D)** Discourse is an aspect of pragmatics that refers to extended language productions in tasks such as conversation and storytelling. Cohesive devices link clausal and sentential elements to form a unified message. Therefore (D) is the correct answer. (A), (B), and (C) are incorrect because they refer to specific aspects of communication that are not related to discourse.

120. **(D)** Intensive phonemic awareness treatment programs are thought to improve reading by training children to differentiate and process speech sounds. However, to date, research has not successfully separated the effects of intensive intervention, so no direct relationship has yet been proven, so (D) is the correct answer. (A), (B), and (C) are incorrect because they address claims about phonemic awareness

treatment that have not been substanti-ated by research.

121. **(A)** is an accurate definition of the speech reception threshold. None of the other answers is accurate. The speech reception threshold is easier to administer than pure-tone audiometry, and it does not use monosyllabic words, so (B) and (C) are incorrect. The speech reception threshold does not measure speech comprehension. Rather, it measures the level at which there is recognition of speech sound, so (D) is incorrect.

122. **(C)** The audiogram depicts a severe to profound hearing loss that is outside the range of speech sounds. Thus, the individual will have difficulty perceiving speech sounds including consonants and vowels, so (C) is the correct answer, and (B) is incorrect. Slurred speech is due to poor muscle control rather than hearing loss, so (A) is incorrect. (D) is incorrect because vocal intensity would be expected to be inconsistently loud and weak.

123. **(D)** Residual hearing at 70 dB in the low frequencies together with hearing levels less than 100 dB at all other frequen-cies suggests a moderately severe to profound hearing loss. Therefore, the correct answer is (D), and (B) and (C) are incorrect. (A) is incorrect because the hearing levels are outside the range for moderate hearing loss.

124. **(B)** Taken together, the first and second formants distinguish most vowel sounds, so (B) is the correct answer. F_3 is not useful for vowel recognition, so (A), (C), and (D) are incorrect.

125. **(A)** Wernicke's aphasia, otherwise known as reception aphasia, is a

disorder of language comprehension and is the result of an infarct to Wernicke's area. Thus, (A) is correct. (B), (C), and (D) are incorrect because infarcts to this area would not result in difficulty in comprehending language.

126. **(D)** Vocal intensity, or loudness, is related to parameters of the oral cavity, lung capacity, and vocal folds, so (A), (B), and (C), are incorrect. (D) is the correct answer because raising of fundamental frequency, or pitch, is unrelated to vocal intensity.

127. **(B)** The symptoms describe chorea, so (B) is the correct answer. (C) and (D) are incorrect because Ballism involves small parts of the body, as in facial tics, and Tourette's syndrome involves concomitant behavior disorders. (A) is incorrect because athetosis is character-ized by slow flowing movements.

128. **(D)** Both apraxia and dysarthria are motor speech disorders caused by damage to the nervous system and both result in articulatory errors, prosodic deficits, and neurological soft signs. Therefore (D) is the correct answer and (A), (B), and (C) are incorrect.

129. **(A)** The protocol employed by the clinician reflects a test-teach-retest sequence known as *dynamic assessment*, so (A) is the correct answer. Functional assessment involves observation in naturalistic contexts, so (B) is incorrect. (C) is incorrect because samples of the child's work are required for portfolio assessment; and (D) is incorrect because authentic assessment occurs outside the clinical environment.

130. **(C)** The correct answer is (C) since the genioglossus is the only extrinsic muscle involved in protrusion of

the tongue. (A) is incorrect since the hyoglossus depresses the tongue. (B) is incorrect because the palatoglossus elevates the back of the tongue and (D) is incorrect because the styloglossus elevates and retracts the tongue.

131. **(C)** Traumatic brain injury results from damage to multiple and diffuse areas of the brain, so (C) is the correct answer. (D) is incorrect because the damage is diffused rather than localized. (A) and (B) are incorrect because they represent specific localized sites.

132. **(D)** The intrinsic laryngeal muscles work synergistically. By its motion, the cricoarytenoid joint serves to abduct and adduct the vocal folds, and the cricothyroid joint lengthens and tenses the vocal folds. Therefore, (D) is the correct answer. (A), (B), and (C) are incorrect because these structures serve different functions.

Score Calculation

Number Correct   _____

Multiplied by 2.65* = _____   **Estimated Praxis Score**

Score Interpretation

162 or Greater	**Excellent!** **You passed**
150–161	**Good** **Practice with test-taking skills is recommended**
149 or Less	**At risk** **Review course material and practice test-taking skills**

*Note that the Praxis may not score all 132 questions and the value of each question may differ from this practice test.

Sources

Questions 1 to 31 from Educational Testing Service (2006, May 25). *The Praxis Series Test Code 0330: Speech-language pathology practice questions* (Chapter 6, pp. 78–83).

Questions 35 to 75 from Educational Testing Service (2006, May 25). *The Praxis Series Test Code 0330: Speech-language pathology practice questions* (Chapter 6, pp. 84–94).

Questions 80 to 121 from Educational Testing Service (2006, May 25). *The Praxis Series Test Code 0330: Speech-language pathology practice questions* (Chapter 6, pp. 94–102).

Appendix C

Coursework Quizzes

There are 19 course quizzes from both the undergraduate and graduate coursework areas represented on the Praxis. Each quiz consists of 10 knowledge and verbatim recall questions to test your basic knowledge. Note that the questions are not Praxis-type questions and that the explanations for the correct and incorrect answers are not provided. The quizzes are designed to reveal your knowledge and recall of information and assess your strengths and weaknesses. Using the Coursework Study Guide in Appendix E, conduct your own research and study to find the correct answers. Based on your score for each quiz, you may need to fully review the course.

Linguistics Quiz

1. In the science of phonology, noticeable changes within the same phoneme class that do not affect meaning or intelligibility are known as:
   A. Phonological errors
   B. Allophones
   C. Phonological processes
   D. Approximations

2. Regular changes to a root word that modify the word's meaning are known as:
   A. Paralinguistic cues
   B. Allophones
   C. Distinctive features
   D. Morphemes

3. Which of the following phonemes may be classified as a diphthong?
   A. /a/ as in father
   B. /aɪ/ as in light
   C. /ɔ/ as in caught
   D. /æ/ as in back

4. Which of the following phoneme classes is produced while the vocal tract is closed or constricted?
   A. Vowels
   B. Consonants
   C. Phonological processes
   D. Allophones

5. Acoustic identification of vowels based on the location of vocal resonance is achieved by examination of:
   A. Formants
   B. Vocal fold vibration
   C. Airflow
   D. Tongue position

6. A dialect is:
   A. A version of a parent language that is uneducated
   B. A mixture of several languages
   C. A subcategory of a parent language
   D. A "broken" variety of a language

7. The rules of language that govern coherence and appropriateness of conversation are known as:

   A. Pragmatic rules
   B. Syntax structure
   C. Paralinguistic cues
   D. Discourse

8. The rule system of language that dictates the combination of the words *it, is,* and *big* to convert a statement to a question is known as:

   A. Transformational rules
   B. Syntactics
   C. Morphemics
   D. Pragmatics

9. Figurative language such as "Don't count your chickens before they hatch" is known as:

   A. Idioms
   B. Metaphors
   C. Proverbs
   D. Similes

10. Which of the following is an example of passive voice?

    A. Tom ate the apples
    B. The apples were eaten by Tom
    C. Tom had eaten the apples
    D. Tom was eating the apples

Language Development Quiz

1. The developmental process in which a young child engages in a long period of producing *consonant-vowel* and *consonant-vowel-consonant* repetitions is known as:

   A. Perseveration
   B. Imitation
   C. Reduplication
   D. Babbling

2. The process of semantic development in which a child acquires the word *climb* while simultaneously increasing her vocabulary through association and adding the words *climber, climbing,* and *climbed* is known as:

   A. Morphology
   B. Fast mapping
   C. Extension
   D. Generalization

3. Which of the following utterances would characterize the holophrastic stage of semantic development?

   A. "Horsie" to refer to a horse
   B. "Cookie" to say "I want a cookie"
   C. "More ball" meaning "throw the ball again"
   D. "Wa wa" meaning "water"

4. Which of the following utterances spoken by a 20-month-old toddler represents the use of "agent + action"?

   A. Doggie eat
   B. Throw it
   C. More juice
   D. Daddy shoe

5. Which of the following is the accurate sequence of the development of consonants?

   A. Velars; palatals; bilabials
   B. Glottals; velars; alveolars
   C. Bilabials; alveolars; glottals
   D. Interdentals; bilabials; alveolars

6. Which of the following phoneme classes is latest to emerge?

   A. Vowels
   B. Nasals
   C. Consonant clusters
   D. Fricatives

7. Which of the following is a phonological process observed in the normal articulation of children 2 to 3 years of age?

A. Liquid simplification
B. Affrication
C. Denasalization
D. Epenthesis

8. A pre-school child who is determined to be in Stage 3 of Brown's Stages of Morphological Development would exhibit a mean length of utterance (MLU) of:
A. 1.5–2.0
B. 2.5–3.0
C. 3.5–3.75
D. 4.0–4.5

9. Which of the following would be classified as a morphological error if observed in the speech of a 3-year-old child?
A. It fall down
B. He do it
C. This a truck
D. I walking

10. A typically developing child should approximate 90% accuracy with adult language by which age range?
A. Preschool
B. School age
C. Early adolescence
D. Late adolescence

Phonetics Quiz

1. Which of the following represents the International Phonetic Alphabet transcription of "language"?
A. /l e g w ɪ j/
B. /l a n g w ɪ dʒ/
C. /l æ n g u æ g/
D. /l e ŋ w ɪ dʒ/

2. Which of the following words does not contain a sibilant phoneme when transcribed in the International Phonetic Alphabet?

A. Ice
B. Church
C. Link
D. Ship

3. Which of the following is classified as a low frontal vowel?
A. /æ/
B. /ʌ/
C. /e/
D. /ɪ/

4. Which of the following words would probably NOT be deciphered without visual cues by an individual with presbycusis?
A. Ghost
B. Watch
C. Gist
D. Joke

5. Which of the following phoneme classes would be affected in an individual with severe velopharyngeal insufficiency?
A. Velars
B. Nasals
C. Glottals
D. Interdentals

6. Which of the following consonants would be difficult to accurately produce for an individual with vocal fold paralysis?
A. /t/
B. /ʃ/
C. /dʒ/
D. /f/

7. Which of the following phonemic pairs would cause confusion for hearing-impaired individuals who rely on speechreading?
A. /f/ and /θ/
B. /l/ and /j/
C. /p/ and /m/
D. /t/ and /k/

8. Consonant production characterized as deaffrication is represented by which of the following?

   A. /dʒ/ → /ʒ/
   B. /t/ → /k/
   C. /d/ → /g/
   D. /z/ → /dʒ/

9. Which of the following sets of phonemes are cognates?

   A. /n/ and /ŋ/
   B. /o/ and /oɪ/
   C. /a/ and /ɔ/
   D. /k/ and /g/

10. Which of the following words contains a semivowel?

   A. Boy
   B. Yes
   C. Hoe
   D. Had

Anatomy and Physiology Quiz

1. During sound production in the larynx, the lowering of pitch is accomplished by the action of which of the following laryngeal muscles?

   A. Thyroarytenoid
   B. Sternohyoid
   C. Thyrohyoid
   D. Cricoarytenoid

2. Muscles of the soft palate include all of the following except:

   A. Genioglossus
   B. Palatoglossus
   C. Palatopharyngeal
   D. Levator veli palatini

3. Which of the following tongue muscles would be predominantly involved in the production of back vowels?

   A. Styloglossus
   B. Hyoglossus
   C. Inferior longitudinal
   D. Palatoglossus

4. If a client is unable to produce plosive sounds, the speech-language pathologist should suspect involvement of which of the following structures of the vocal tract?

   A. Tongue
   B. Nares
   C. Lips
   D. Uvula

5. During the oral phase of swallowing when the bolus is transferred to the pharynx, an important function to prevent the bolus from entering the larynx is accomplished by the:

   A. Tongue
   B. Velum
   C. Epiglottis
   D. Esophagus

6. The fifth cranial nerve, which is essential to speech, is also known as:

   A. Facial
   B. Trigeminal
   C. Vagus
   D. Abducens

7. Which of the following is not a muscle of inspiration?

   A. Internal intercostal
   B. Diaphragm
   C. Abdomen
   D. Sternocleidomastoid

8. Which of the following is not a structure involved in transforming sound waves to neural impulses?

   A. Tympanic membrane
   B. Eustacean tube
   C. Stapedius muscle
   D. Semicircular canals

9. Which of the following is not a structure contained in the inner ear?

   A. Basilar membrane
   B. Tympanic membrane
   C. Cochlea
   D. Organ of Corti

10. Which lobe of the brain is associated with hearing function?

   A. Frontal
   B. Temporal
   C. Occipital
   D. Parietal

Diagnostic Methods Quiz

1. Which of the following is not true with regard to standardized language tests?

   A. Scores are based on performance of a normative sample
   B. Several parameters of language behaviors are probed
   C. There is a strict protocol for administration
   D. Outcomes suggest specific targets for treatment

2. Etiology of a disorder may be inferred from

   A. Case history
   B. Observed behaviors during assessment
   C. Performance profile on a standard-ized test
   D. Performance on a battery of diag-nostic procedures

3. Which of the following clinical services may not be conducted by a speech-language pathologist with clients with a suspected hearing loss?

   A. Pure-tone audiometry battery
   B. Screening air conduction thresholds
   C. Otoscopic inspection
   D. Screening tympanometry

4. Which of the following is an example of a "Cloze" item on a language test?

   A. "Say cat"
   B. "Point to the big red ball"
   C. "Show me the cow"
   D. "Here is a bird. Here are two ____"

5. In assessment of linguistics skills, mean length of utterance (MLU) is a measure of:

   A. Semantic development
   B. Morphological development
   C. Phrase structure
   D. Sentence comprehension

6. Which of the following activities distinguishes dynamic assessment from traditional assessment procedures?

   A. Qualitative analysis
   B. Language sampling
   C. Test-teach-retest process
   D. Alternate scoring process

7. In language sample scoring, the type-token ratio is a measure of:

   A. Syntactic development
   B. Semantic development
   C. Morphological development
   D. Pragmatic development

8. The number of morphemes in the sentence "Mommy gives good hugs" is:

   A. 3
   B. 4
   C. 5
   D. 6

9. Which of the following is a compre-hensive inventory that assesses communicative skills as well as social and motor skills in infants and toddlers?

   A. Preschool Language Scale
   B. Bayley Scales of Infant Development
   C. Vineland Adaptive Behavior Scales
   D. Battelle Development Inventory

10. A clinician conducts an evaluation of a client who has sustained a cerebrovascular accident. Which of the following is not typically a measure conducted during the evaluation?

    A. Determining the severity of language impairment
    B. Locating the site of the lesion
    C. Formulating a prognosis for recovery
    D. Identifying the characteristics of language disorder

Clinical Methods Quiz

1. Which of the following is the accurate sequence in the treatment of communication behaviors?

    A. Fading; elicitation; generalization; maintenance
    B. Fading; elicitation, maintenance; generalization
    C. Elicitation; fading; maintenance; generalization
    D. Elicitation; maintenance; generalization; fading

2. A clinician provides treatment for a client who stutters using a token economy. For every occurrence of a stuttering behavior, the clinician withdraws one token from the client. This type of reinforcement protocol is known as:

    A. Punishment
    B. Negative reinforcement
    C. Fading
    D. Contingency reinforcement

3. A clinician provides treatment for a client who stutters. A continuous mild intrusive crackling sound ceases whenever the client maintains fluency. This behavior management protocol is known as:

    A. Response shaping
    B. Token economy

    C. Negative reinforcement
    D. Positive reinforcement

4. A major disadvantage of standardized tests in the differential diagnosis of a communication disorders is:

    A. Standardized tests lack content validity
    B. Standardized tests lack reliability
    C. Standardized tests are based on a limited norming sample
    D. Standardized tests do not probe the all parameters of the behavior

5. In the pretreatment phase of intervention for a communication disorder, a clinician obtains a baseline to:

    A. Measure the severity of the disorder
    B. Obtain data for gauging progress
    C. Formulate a prognosis for recovery
    D. Prioritize treatment goals

6. Which of the following is an appropriate statement of a treatment objective?

    A. Colin will correctly answer 8 out of 10 wh-questions
    B. By the end of the treatment session Colin will correctly answer 10 wh-questions with 80% accuracy
    C. By the end of the treatment session Colin will be able to answer wh-questions
    D. Colin will improve his ability to answer wh-questions

7. Which of the following is an appropriate Individualized Education Plan (IEP) goal for a child with autism spectrum disorder?

    A. Mary will improve social communication skills by the end of the first advisory
    B. Mary will initiate communication with peers in the classroom
    C. Mary will understand specific social communication behaviors (i.e., turn-taking, body language) when required in group treatment sessions

D. By the end of the treatment session Mary will correctly identify communication breakdowns and make appropriate modifications in 4 out of 5 trials

8. During treatment procedures, a probe is:

   A. A stimulus provided by the clinician to elicit a response from the client
   B. A measurement taken by the clinician following a treatment activity
   C. A stimulus provided by the clinician that is not one of the target behaviors
   D. A measurement taken by the clinician to assess progress

9. Evidence from the research suggests that the most effective treatment contingency to increase a desired behavior is:

   A. A fixed reinforcement schedule
   B. A random reinforcement schedule
   C. A continuous reinforcement schedule
   D. An intermittent reinforcement schedule

10. Response generalization refers to:

    A. Carryover
    B. Maintenance
    C. Mastery
    D. New behaviors

Audiology Quiz

1. Which of the following audiologic results would indicate a sensorineural hearing loss?

   A. Both air conduction and bone conduction thresholds are decreased, but bone conduction exceeds air conduction
   B. Both air conduction and bone conduction are decreased in higher frequencies

   C. Air conduction thresholds exceed bone conduction
   D. Both thresholds are decreased, and air conduction and bone conduction thresholds are equivalent

2. On the standard pure-tone audiogram, "hertz" and "dB" refer to which of the following?

   A. Frequency and sound pressure level
   B. Frequency and hearing level
   C. Hearing level and frequency
   D. Hearing level and sound pressure level

3. A disease involving the bony capsule of the inner ear that manifests in a conductive hearing loss is:

   A. Otitis media
   B. Otosclerosis
   C. Tinnitus
   D. Mastoiditis

4. Which of the following is not a bone in the middle ear?

   A. Mastoid
   B. Malleus
   C. Incus
   D. Stapes

5. A frequency not included in the "speech banana" of the standard pure-tone audiogram is:

   A. 5000
   B. 6000
   C. 7000
   D. 8000

6. Which of the following will be evident in the audiogram of an individual with otitis media?

   A. Decreased threshold levels for high frequencies
   B. Decreased threshold levels at all frequencies
   C. Air-bone gap
   D. Carhart notch

7. A hearing loss at 71–90 dB is categorized as:

    A. Mild
    B. Moderate
    C. Severe
    D. Profound

8. Which of the following conditions would yield a Type B (flat) tympanogram?

    A. Otosclerosis
    B. Tympanic membrane perforation
    C. Acoustic neuroma
    D. Otitis media

9. Which of the following causes of hearing loss is not associated with the middle ear?

    A. Acoustic tumor
    B. Cholesteotoma
    C. Otosclerosis
    D. Otitis media

10. With regard to identification of individuals with hearing impairment, under the ASHA Scope of Practice, a speech-language pathologist may conduct:

    A. Impedance testing
    B. Pure-tone audiological screening
    C. Pure-tone audiological testing
    D. Speech audiometry

Neuroanatomy/ Neurophysiology Quiz

1. A client exhibits symptoms of impaired sensitivity and mobility of the tongue, lips, and oral structures, and delayed swallow reflex due to a mild brainstem stroke. Given the symptoms and general location of the infarct, which of the following cranial nerves are most probably affected?

    A. Vagus; hypoglossal; glossopharyngeal
    B. Facial; hypoglossal; glossopharyngeal
    C. Trigeminal; vagus; hypoglossal
    D. Trigeminal; facial; vagus

2. Upon request to protrude the tongue, which of the following neurological soft signs if observed in a 78-year-old adult would indicate a lesion to upper motor neurons in the left hemisphere?

    A. Tongue deviation to the right side
    B. Tongue deviation to the left side
    C. Inability to protrude the tongue
    D. Lack of tongue strength

3. Which of the following areas of the cerebral cortex is least involved in speech production?

    A. Premotor cortex
    B. Sensorimotor cortex
    C. Broca's area
    D. Wernicke's area

4. A lesion to the brainstem involving the medulla oblongata would result in deficits in:

    A. Mastication
    B. Coordination
    C. Swallowing
    D. Tongue protrusion

5. Disturbances of muscular control related to coordination of speech movements result from damage to the:

    A. Cerebellum
    B. Motor cortex
    C. Cranial nerves
    D. Pons

6. Which of the following is a cranial nerve that is both sensory and motor:

    A. Abducens
    B. Acoustic
    C. Facial
    D. Vagus

7. Contraction of the levator veli palatini muscle is innervated by which of the following cranial nerves?

   A. Glossopharyngeal
   B. Vagus
   C. Trigeminal
   D. Abducens

8. Disconnection syndrome would result from a lesion to which of the following?

   A. Spinal cord
   B. Central nervous system
   C. Peripheral nervous system
   D. Corpus collosum

9. Left side neglect is symptomatic of a lesion to the:

   A. Left frontal-parietal lobe
   B. Right frontal-parietal lobe
   C. Optic nerve
   D. Oculomotor nerve

10. A lesion to the hippocampus would result in impaired:

    A. Short-term memory
    B. Long-term memory
    C. Speech production
    D. Visual agnosia

Articulation Disorders Quiz

1. A child who exhibits the phonological process of fronting would produce which of the following?

   A. /gjo/ for "go"
   B. /gagi/ for "doggie"
   C. /wæbɪt/ for "rabbit"
   D. /tæt/ for "cat"

2. In normal pronunciation, which of the following might be rendered with weak syllable deletion?

   A. Always
   B. Valley
   C. About
   D. Argue

3. Which of the following pairs are linguistic cognates?

   A. "Size" and "lies"
   B. "Seal" and "zeal"
   C. "Cat" and "bat"
   D. "Fish" and "wish"

4. In selection of target sounds for intervention with a child with an articulation disorder, the clinician would most appropriately begin treatment with phonemes that are:

   A. Stimulable
   B. Earliest acquired
   C. Most critical to intelligibility
   D. Most visible in place and manner of articulation

5. Which approach to treatment of a phonological disorder emphasizes modeling, visualizing, and recasting of a longer utterance rather than focusing on a target phoneme in isolation?

   A. Morphosyntax approach
   B. Whole language approach
   C. Core vocabulary approach
   D. Metaphonological approach

6. After assessment it is determined that most of a child's articulation errors are distortions related to imprecise placement and lack of coordination in motor skills. An appropriate treatment method is:

   A. Distinctive Feature approach
   B. Metaphon Therapy approach
   C. Cycles Remediation approach
   D. Sensory-Motor approach\

7. For a child with velopharyngeal insufficiency, which of the following is the most appropriate treatment goal?

   A. Oral motor exercises to increase strength and mobility
   B. Compensatory articulatory strategies
   C. Alternative communication device
   D. Esophageal speech

8. In evaluation of a speech sample, phonological mean length of utterance relates to:

   A. Patterns of errors
   B. Randomness of errors
   C. Frequency of errors
   D. Intelligibility

9. In the progress of treatment for speech sound disorders, generalization would be expected:

   A. Automatically as a result of treatment
   B. For phonemes in the same response class
   C. Across minimal pairs
   D. As a phonological process is addressed

10. A theory of phonological disorders that posits that errors arise from faulty perceptual skills and that focuses treatment on ear training is known as:

    A. Structural theory
    B. Generative Phonology theory
    C. McDonald Sensory-Motor approach
    D. Van Riper's Traditional approach

Language Disorders Quiz

1. The intervention method for a child with a language disorder in which the clinician comments on actions simultaneously as they are performed such as "I'm coloring my ball blue" is known as:

   A. Reauditorization
   B. Self-talk
   C. Recasting
   D. Parallel talk

2. The language teaching process in which the clinician presents a stimulus and elicits a verbal response and then presents a reinforcement is known as:

   A. Joint action routine
   B. Direct teaching
   C. Incidental teaching
   D. Milieu intervention

3. Which of the following standardized measures of language skills examines both receptive and expressive language?

   A. Peabody Picture Vocabulary Test
   B. Clinical Evaluation of Language Skills
   C. WORD Test
   D. Boehm Test of Basic Concepts

4. Intervention for children who exhibit high-functioning autism would most likely focus on:

   A. Vocabulary development
   B. Receptive language
   C. Expressive language
   D. Pragmatic skills

5. Alternatives to standardized testing include all of the following except:

   A. Dynamic assessment
   B. Narrative assessment
   C. Criterion referenced testing
   D. Intelligence testing

6. Language assessment for prelinguistic infants and toddlers may utilize which of the following?

   A. Symbolic play
   B. Imitation routines
   C. Social behaviors
   D. Developmental milestones

7. For calculating the mean length of utterance (MLU) for the following language sample, "Bobby's friend dropped his glasses while he was running," the total morphemic count is:

   A. 9
   B. 12
   C. 13
   D. 15

8. A clinician who utilizes emojis and emoticons as stimuli in instruction to a child with autism is most likely employing which treatment strategy?

   A. Applied Behavior Analysis
   B. Theory of Mind
   C. Floor Time
   D. Picture Exchange Communication

9. Higher-order cognitive skills involved in reading comprehension include all of the following except:

   A. Planning
   B. Drawing inferences
   C. Imagery
   D. Concluding

10. Which of the following is not typically an etiological factor related to intellectual ability?

   A. Lead poisoning
   B. Socioeconomic status
   C. Low birth weight
   D. Ethnic background

Stuttering Quiz

1. Which of the following statements represents the continuity hypothesis of the etiology of stuttering?

   A. Stuttering symptoms develop in adolescence
   B. Presence of family history of stuttering

   C. Stuttering occurs in predictable elements of the speech utterance
   D. Stuttering behavior is preceded by normal child dysfluency

2. Early characteristics of normal nonfluent speech by preschool children may be characterized by:

   A. Sound and syllable repetitions
   B. Word and phrase repetitions
   C. Sound prolongations
   D. Tension while speaking

3. Adherence to the Diagnosogenic-Semantic theory of stuttering would lead to which of the following treatment strategies?

   A. Fluency shaping
   B. Environmental manipulation
   C. Client and family counseling
   D. Desensitization therapy

4. The fact that some individuals who stutter achieve complete fluency while singing is explained by which of the following theories of etiology?

   A. Neuropsycholinguistic
   B. Laryngeal dysfunction
   C. Anticipatory struggle
   D. Psychoneurosis

5. Measurement of stuttering severity includes which of the following procedures?

   A. Respiratory dynamics
   B. Laryngeal dynamics
   C. Articulatory dynamics
   D. Duration of struggle behavior

6. Technology-based treatment of stuttering through fluency shaping includes which of the following techniques?

   A. Delayed auditory feedback
   B. Continuous phonation
   C. Prolonged speech
   D. Rate reduction

7. Which of the following statements regarding the adaptation effect is FALSE?

   A. The adaptation effect is a temporary phenomenon
   B. Rehearsal by reading silently before oral reading produces greater adaptation
   C. Some individuals exhibit increased stuttering rather than adaptation effect
   D. Adaptation is associated with reduction of fear

8. A clinician observes that on repeated oral readings of the same passage, a client stutters on the words *me* and *and* 100% of the time. This phenomenon is known as:

   A. Adjacency effect
   B. Adjustment effect
   C. Consistency effect
   D. Adaptation effect

9. Behaviors exhibited by a client during stuttering including eye blinking, facial tics, and head bobbing are known as:

   A. Compensatory strategies
   B. Prompts
   C. Secondary behaviors
   D. Anticipatory struggles

10. Which of the following is the most important diagnostic indicator for the distinction of developmental dysfluency and stuttering in preschool children?

   A. Whole-word repetitions
   B. Sound repetitions
   C. Phrase repetitions
   D. Familial history of stuttering

Voice Disorders Quiz

1. Which of the following maneuvers would be required in order to lower fundamental frequency in a client whose vocal pitch is too high?

   A. Lengthening and thickening the vocal folds
   B. Shortening and thinning the vocal folds
   C. Elevating the larynx in the throat
   D. Decreasing tracheal airflow

2. A clinician treats an individual with weak breathy vocal quality due to dysarthria. Treatment for vocal quality should be targeted at:

   A. Strengthening extrinsic laryngeal musculature
   B. Strengthening articulatory musculature
   C. Raising fundamental frequency
   D. Increasing subglottal air pressure

3. The vocal quality characterized by a low pitch and crackly voice is known as:

   A. Stridency
   B. Vocal fry
   C. Harshness
   D. Hoarseness

4. Sound production for esophageal speech is effectuated by which of the following laryngeal muscles?

   A. Stylopharyngeus
   B. Cricopharyngeal
   C. Palatopharyngeus
   D. Levator veli palatini

5. A client with a papilloma will experience all of the following symptoms except:

   A. Low pitch
   B. Hoarseness
   C. Breathiness
   D. Pitch break

6. Which of the following is not a treatment technique for reducing vocal hyperfunction with a client with a voice disorders due to vocal abuse?

A. Yawn-sigh
B. Gentle onset
C. Chewing approach
D. Pushing

7. A surgically implanted prosthetic device that becomes a sound source for individuals with a laryngectomy is:
A. Blom-Singer
B. Nasometer
C. Endoscope
D. Layrngoscope

8. The s/z ratio is a measurement of:
A. Respiratory capacity
B. Oral resonance
C. Phonatory adequacy
D. Vocal fold vibration

9. Damage to which of the following cranial nerves would produce aphonia?
A. Trigeminal
B. Vagus
C. Glossopharyngeal
D. Hypoglossal

10. A woman who is an entertainer and singer with symptoms including hoarseness, breathiness, and a feeling of a lump inside the throat consults a speech-language pathologist. Prior to initiation of treatment the client should be referred to the otolaryngologist to rule out:
A. Spasmodic dysphonia
B. Vocal fold paralysis
C. Vocal fold polyp
D. Laryngeal web

Augmentative/Alternative Communication (AAC) Quiz

1. A speech-generating device is an example of:

A. An unaided device
B. A PECS system
C. A high-tech aided device
D. A low-tech aided device

2. A temporary AAC system would be recommended for an individual with which of the following conditions?
A. Laryngectomy
B. Cerebral palsy
C. Vocal nodules
D. Vocal fold paralysis

3. Which of the following is an example of direct selection for an individual using an augmentative speech device?
A. Eye gaze
B. Auditory scanning
C. Sip and puff
D. Inverse switch

4. Which of the following has the highest level of iconicity?
A. ASL symbol
B. Blissymbol
C. Print word
D. Rebus

5. Which of the following is not a technique for timing enhancement in the production of written messages?
A. Word prediction
B. Alpha word code
C. QWERTY layout
D. Abbreviation expansion

6. In the selection of a speech generating device, the advantage of digitized speech over synthesized speech is:
A. Ease of retrieval
B. Fidelity of the signal
C. Memory capacity for messaging
D. Natural sound quality

7. Which of the following is the most important factor in selection of a low-tech device over a high-tech device?

   A. Funding
   B. Cognitive ability
   C. Visual acuity
   D. Motor ability

8. A scanning method where the user ceases activation of a switch when the desired symbol is reached is known as:

   A. Circular scanning
   B. Linear scanning
   C. Group-item scanning
   D. Step scanning

9. Which of the following is not a typical method for rate enhancement for message formulation and transmission in a user of an augmentative communication device?

   A. Partner-assisted scanning
   B. Alphanumeric coding
   C. Word prediction
   D. Color coding

10. The vocabulary inventory for the user of an augmentative communication device should be appropriate for which of the following?

    A. High-frequency words
    B. New words not in the user's vocabulary
    C. Age
    D. All of the above

Neurogenic Language Disorders Quiz

1. A type of aphasia characterized by intact comprehension but presence of echolalia, perseveration, and reduced spontaneous speech is:

   A. Global aphasia
   B. Transcortical motor aphasia
   C. Broca's aphasia
   D. Wernicke's aphasia

2. The type of aphasia that generally affects auditory comprehension is:

   A. Anomic aphasia
   B. Conduction aphasia
   C. Broca's aphasia
   D. Wernicke's aphasia

3. A disruption to blood flow in the middle cerebral artery is most likely to result in which type of aphasia?

   A. Transcortical sensory aphasia
   B. Transcortical motor aphasia
   C. Anomic aphasia
   D. Global aphasia

4. Problems in comprehending nonliteral and figurative language are generally associated with:

   A. Normal aging
   B. Sensory aphasia
   C. Right hemisphere brain damage
   D. Conduction aphasia

5. A client exhibits right hemisphere hemiplegia in addition to characteristics of aphasia. The speech-language pathologist may infer that the site of lesion is in the:

   A. Left hemisphere
   B. Right hemisphere
   C. Frontal lobe
   D. Temporal lobe

6. An individual with which of the following types of aphasia will be an appropriate candidate for Melodic Intonation Therapy?

   A. Broca's aphasia
   B. Wernicke's aphasia
   C. Conduction aphasia
   D. Anomic aphasia

7. Melodic Intonation Therapy is designed to improve:

   A. Auditory comprehension
   B. Word recognition
   C. Sentence production
   D. Production of single words

8. An environment-based treatment for aphasia that emphasizes training of the client's conversation partner is:

   A. Visual Action Therapy
   B. Treatment of Underlying Forms
   C. Supported Conversation for Adults
   D. Melodic Intonation Therapy

9. Which of the following is not a prognostic indicator for recovery of language function for a client with aphasia?

   A. Onset of treatment
   B. Type of aphasia
   C. Site of lesion
   D. Education

10. A clinician who administers the ASHA-FACS to a client with aphasia is examining:

    A. Auditory comprehension
    B. Functional communication
    C. Syntactic ability
    D. Cognitive function

Swallowing Disorders Quiz

1. Damage to which of the following cranial nerves will affect the ability to achieve a complete seal in the early stages of swallowing?

   A. Facial
   B. Trigeminal
   C. Hypoglossal
   D. Abducens

2. Which of the following is a valve that opens during the pharyngeal phase of the swallowing process?

   A. Aryepiglottic folds
   B. Vocal folds
   C. Upper esophageal sphincter
   D. Velopharynx

3. Which of the following procedures would provide the most complete information regarding all the phases of the swallowing proves?

   A. Modified barium swallow
   B. Electromyography
   C. Ultrasound
   D. Endoscopy

4. Movements during which of the following phase(s) of the swallowing process are reflexive?

   A. Oral preparatory and oral
   B. Oral and pharyngeal
   C. Pharyngeal and esophageal
   D. Esophageal

5. The greatest possibility for aspiration into the lungs occurs during which of the following phases of the swallow?

   A. Oral preparatory
   B. Oral
   C. Pharyngeal
   D. Transitional

6. A treatment procedure in which stimulation is presented to the faucial pillars to affect the swallow reflex is known as:

   A. Thermal stimulation
   B. Palatal reshaping
   C. Postural adjustment
   D. Oromotor swallow exercise

7. The primary goal of dysphagia treatment is to:

   A. Prevent aspiration
   B. Ensure adequate nutritional status
   C. Repair swallow function
   D. Teach compensatory swallow behaviors

8. Individuals with which of the following conditions have the best prognosis for recovery of swallowing function?
   A. Parkinson's disease
   B. Myasthenia gravis
   C. Muscular dystrophy
   D. Unilateral hemisphere stroke

9. Treatment using the Mendelsohn maneuver would be best suited to an individual with which of the following difficulties?
   A. Delayed swallow reflex
   B. Elevating the tongue
   C. Elevating the larynx
   D. Vocal fold closure

10. A modified barium swallow revealed evidence of pooling thin liquids in the valleculae. This most likely occurred during which of the following phases of the swallow?
    A. Pharyngeal
    B. Transitional
    C. Esophageal
    D. Oral

Motor Speech Disorders Quiz

1. Hypernasality is a common speech characteristic associated with which of the following?
   A. Apraxia
   B. Parkinson's disease
   C. Aphasia
   D. Bulbar paralysis

2. Which of the following is not affected in dysarthria?
   A. Phonation
   B. Language

C. Resonance
D. Prosody

3. An 80-year-old man has been referred to a speech-language pathologist after his admission to the hospital following a mild stroke. Speech examination reveals muscle weakness and lack of muscular control. The client's diagnosis should indicate:
   A. Ataxic dysarthria
   B. Hyperkinetic dysarthria
   C. Hypokinetic dysarthria
   D. Flaccid dysarthria

4. A 6-year-old child has numerous articulatory errors accompanied by uncoordinated positioning of the lips and tongue and slow, labored speech. The speech-language pathologist's treatment plan should be initiated with:
   A. Oral positioning of consonant sounds
   B. Speech sounds acquired earliest
   C. Consonant/vowel and vowel/consonant syllables
   D. Improvement of prosody

5. Which of the following is not a prognostic indicator for recovery from apraxia?
   A. Etiology
   B. Severity
   C. Time of onset
   D. Premorbid language ability

6. Which of the following would be a result of damage to the cerebellum?
   A. Flaccid dysarthria
   B. Ataxic dysarthria
   C. Spastic dysarthria
   D. Apraxia

7. Treatment for dysarthria would appropriately proceed with the following as an initial goal:

A. Improving speech rate
B. Training compensatory articulatory movements
C. Instruction in the use of an alternative communication device
D. Establishing respiratory support for speech production

8. A client exhibits variability in the production of /f/ in the following sentence, "Floyd could not faithfully fulfill his functions." The most probable diagnosis is:
A. Hypokinesis
B. Apraxia
C. Ataxia
D. Dysarthria

9. Which of the following functions would not be affected in a client with ataxic dysarthria?
A. Swallowing difficulty
B. Articulatory inaccuracy
C. Phonatory impairment
D. Prosodic disturbance

10. Due to the effect of decreased motor control, the speech characteristics of which of the following types of dysarthria most resemble apraxia?
A. Hypokinetic dysarthria
B. Hyperkinetic dysarthria
C. Ataxic dysarthria
D. Spastic dysarthria

Traumatic Brain Injury Quiz

1. Which of the following is an important indicator in the prognosis for recovery in traumatic brain injury?
A. Performance on standardized measures
B. Residual memory

C. Attention and concentration ability
D. Length of time in a coma

2. A communication behavior presented in individuals with traumatic brain injury that distinguishes traumatic brain injury from aphasia is:
A. Confabulations
B. Irritability
C. Perseveration
D. Naming difficulties

3. An individual with traumatic brain injury may exhibit difficulty in maintaining topic in conversation, turn-taking, rambling speech, and confused language. The speech-language pathologist should initiate treatment for:
A. Pragmatic language problems
B. Cognitive rehabilitation
C. Attention and concentration
D. Organizational skills

4. A communication behavior common to traumatic brain injury and neurological disorders is:
A. Aphasia
B. Dysarthria
C. Apraxia
D. Right hemisphere syndrome

5. The leading cause of traumatic brain injuries is:
A. Car accidents
B. Falls
C. Pedestrian accidents
D. Sports injuries

6. The group most susceptible to traumatic brain injuries is:
A. Children
B. Elderly
C. Females
D. Males

7. The state of an individual who is awake and aware of his/her surroundings and who can communicate with eye blinks but not speech is:

   A. Vegetative
   B. Locked-in syndrome
   C. Comatose
   D. Semi-comatose

8. An individual who suffered a traumatic brain injury exhibits visual agnosia. This problem is most likely due to injury in which area of the brain?

   A. Parietal lobe
   B. Frontal lobe
   C. Occipital lobe
   D. Temporal lobe

9. A brain injury that results in a blood clot outside the blood vessels is known as:

   A. Hemorrhage
   B. Edema
   C. Hematoma
   D. Concussion

10. An individual with traumatic brain injury experiences emotional and personality problems as well as problems in cognition, planning, and organizing. These problems are most probably related to injuries in the:

    A. Parietal lobe
    B. Motor cortex
    C. Frontal lobe
    D. Temporal lobe

Research Methods Quiz

1. An investigator conducts an experimental study in which the test scores of a group of participants on a pretest given before a treatment session are compared to a post-test given after treatment. The treatment is designed to increase their scores; however, statistical analysis reveals no significant differences in the means for the two tests. In this situation the investigator must:

   A. Reject the null hypothesis
   B. Accept the null hypothesis
   C. Replicate the experimental procedures with a different group
   D. Modify the post-test

2. In a research investigation, Version A of a test instrument is administered to a group of 30 participants. Two weeks later, Version B of the same instrument is administered, and the results are compared for each participant. No significant differences in the scores of Version A and B are observed. The investigator may conclude:

   A. There is validity of Version A
   B. There is validity of Version B
   C. There is validity of both versions
   D. There is reliability between the two versions

3. Which of the following is a measure of dispersion among scores?

   A. Standard deviation
   B. Mean
   C. Mode
   D. Median

4. In relation to the normal curve, a left-skewed distribution indicates:

   A. Fewer scores lower than the mean
   B. A greater number of scores lower than the mean
   C. A very low mean
   D. A very high mean

5. An investigator gathers data from a large sample of individuals with hearing loss. The thresholds are recorded and classified as either a mild, moderate, severe, or profound hearing loss. The type of data represented by the classification of scores is known as:

A. Interval
B. Ratio
C. Continuous
D. Nominal

6. In an experimental study, "control" relates to the process of:

A. Equalizing the number of participants in each group
B. Utilizing measures that are reliable and valid
C. Minimizing the effect of extraneous variables
D. Measuring the independent variable

7. The results of a developmental investigation reveal that as children advance in age, the frequency of disfluencies in their speech decreases. With regard to the relationship between age and disfluency, these findings permit which of the following conclusions?

A. Cause-effect
B. Predictive
C. Positive correlation
D. Negative correlation

8. An investigator hypothesizes a relationship between birth order and presence of autism in children. The most appropriate research design to investigate this hypothesis is:

A. Experimental
B. Correlational
C. Survey
D. Cross-sectional

9. In a research study to examine the effect of the loudness of concert music on the duration of temporary hearing threshold shifts in young adults, the independent variable is:

A. Loudness
B. Age
C. Hearing level
D. Onset of threshold shift

10. In a research study to examine the effect of the loudness of concert music on the duration of temporary hearing threshold shift in young adults, the dependent variable is:

A. Age
B. dB level
C. Hearing level
D. Duration of threshold shift

Multicultural Issues Quiz

1. The variety of English spoken by an individual who acquired English as a second language may manifest permanent influences from the native language. This phenomenon is known as:

A. Dialect
B. Speech disorder
C. Accent
D. Broken English

2. A 5-year-old child is developing linguistic skills in two languages. She is referred to a speech-language pathologist because she often mixes words from both languages within the same sentence. This normal developmental process is known as:

A. Semilingualism
B. Sequential bilingualism
C. Code switching
D. Fossilization

3. Which of the following would be a false negative if scored as incorrect on a standardized test for a 4-year-old child developing African-American English?

A. I go to kool
B. I have two pencil
C. That John book
D. She nice

4. On a test of syntax, which of the following would be a true error rather than a language influence for a 5-year-old bilingual Spanish-speaking child?

   A. What this is?
   B. Juan no have none
   C. I'm more tall
   D. No more the music

5. Which of the following is a true statement regarding a linguistic dialect?

   A. Dialects are spoken by uneducated populations
   B. Everyone speaks a dialect
   C. Dialects emerge from misuse of a language
   D. A dialect is a nonstandard variety of a language

6. Which of the following is a type of bias found in some standardized tests in which a child is unfamiliar with the performance expectations of the test due to cultural difference?

   A. Examiner bias
   B. Pragmatic bias
   C. Social/situational bias
   D. Directions/format bias

7. Which of the following is not an alternative method of assessment to avoid test bias in standardized tests?

   A. Qualitative assessment
   B. Dynamic assessment
   C. Alternative scoring
   D. Ethnographic interview

8. Which of the following is the LEAST appropriate alternative to be used by a clinician when no language test is available in a child's native language?

   A. Utilize a translator
   B. Translate the test
   C. Administer the items in both languages
   D. Dynamic assessment

9. For assessment of bilingual children, the native language is defined as:

   A. The language in which the child is most proficient
   B. The language used by the child's parents
   C. The language used in the home
   D. The language of the country of origin

10. Which of the following is not a typical behavior in second-language acquisition that, if observed in a client, may indicate the presence of a disorder?

    A. Language loss of the first language
    B. Language mixing between languages
    C. Silent period when both languages are seldom used
    D. Arrested development of both languages

Answers to Coursework Quizzes

Linguistics Quiz

1. B 2. D 3. B 4. B 5. A 6. C 7. A 8. B 9. C 10. B Score ____%

Language Development Quiz

1. D 2. B 3. B 4. A 5. C 6. C 7. A 8. B 9. D 10. C Score ____%

Phonetics Quiz

1. D 2. C 3. A 4. C 5. B 6. B 7. C 8. A 9. D 10. B Score ____%

Anatomy and Physiology Quiz

1. B 2. A 3. D 4. C 5. C 6. B 7. C 8. D 9. B 10. B Score ____%

Clinical Methods Quiz

1. C 2. A 3. C 4. D 5. B 6. B 7. D 8. C 9. D 10. A Score ____%

Diagnostic Methods Quiz

1. D 2. A 3. A 4. D 5. B 6. C 7. B 8. D 9. C 10. B Score ____%

Audiology Quiz

1. D 2. B 3. B 4. A 5. D 6. C 7. C 8. D 9. A 10. B Score ____%

Neuroanatomy/Neurophysiology Quiz

1. A 2. A 3. D 4. C 5. A 6. D 7. B 8. D 9. B 10. A Score ____%

Articulation Disorders Quiz

1. D 2. C 3. B 4. A 5. B 6. D 7. B 8. C 9. B 10. D Score ____%

Language Disorders Quiz

1. D 2. B 3. B 4. D 5. D 6. D 7. B 8. B 9. A 10. D Score ____%

Stuttering Quiz

1. D 2. B 3. D 4. A 5. D 6. A 7. B 8. C 9. C 10. D Score ____%

Voice Disorders Quiz

1. A 2. D 3. B 4. B 5. D 6. D 7. A 8. C 9. B 10. C Score ____%

Augmentative/Alternative Communication (AAC) Quiz

1. C 2. C 3. A 4. D 5. C 6. B 7. C 8. D 9. A 10. D Score ____%

Neurogenic Language Disorders Quiz

1. B 2. D 3. A 4. C 5. A 6. A 7. C 8. C 9. D 10. B Score ____%

Swallowing Disorders Quiz

1. B 2. C 3. A 4. C 5. D 6. A 7. B 8. D 9. C 10. A Score ____%

Motor Speech Disorders Quiz

1. D 2. B 3. D 4. A 5. D 6. B 7. D 8. B 9. A 10. C Score ____%

Traumatic Brain Injury Quiz

1. D 2. C 3. A 4. B 5. B 6. D 7. B 8. C 9. C 10. C Score ____%

Research Methods Quiz

1. B 2. D 3. A 4. A 5. D 6. C 7. D 8. B 9. A 10. D Score ____%

Multicultural Issues Quiz

1. C 2. C 3. A 4. D 5. B 6. C 7. A 8. B 9. C 10. D Score ____%

Coursework Study Guide

Questions on the Praxis are designed to assess course knowledge, but more importantly, the application of course knowledge to clinical situations. You should expect few questions on basic facts (e.g., definitions, etiology) and few verbatim recall questions. Most Praxis questions require clinical decision making based on information about the disorders, their diagnoses, and treatment. The present Coursework Study Guide lists what you should know for the Praxis and directs you to suggested sources for review of course information.

The Praxis covers information from undergraduate and graduate courses, categorized as: (a) Foundations and Professional Practice; (b) Screening, Assessment, Evaluation, and Diagnosis; and (c) Planning, Implementation and Evaluation of Treatment which are further described on the Educational Testing Service (ETS) website. For each of these areas, this book lists the most important concepts to know from 18 undergraduate and graduate courses. In addition, a sample Praxis question is provided for each coursework area to help you identify and utilize the reasoning skills discussed in Chapter 4.

First, take the coursework quizzes in Appendix D to identify areas of weakness. But don't limit your study to areas of weakness and don't study to memorize facts since it is most important to understand how the course information informs clinical decisions.

Linguistics

Praxis Area 1: Foundations

I. Terminology and Concepts
   Allophone, Cognate, Deep/Surface structure, Derivational/Inflectional morphology, Dialect, Discourse, Distinctive feature, Form/Content/Use, Idiom, Lexicon, Linguistic competence/Performance, Metalinguistics, Minimal pair, Morpheme/Morphology, Noun/Verb phrase, Parts of speech, Phoneme/Phonology, Pragmatics, Prosody, Semantic/Syntactic ambiguity, Syntax, Tree diagram

II. **Elements of Language**
   A. Phonology
      1. Speech sounds; International Phonetic Alphabet (IPA)
      2. Phoneme classes: vowels, consonants, distinctive features
      3. Phoneme production: place, manner, resonance
   B. Semantics/Morphology
      1. Semantic features, root words, bound and free morphemes
      2. Morphological processes: derivational and inflectional morphology
      3. Idioms, semantic ambiguity
   C. Syntax
      1. Parts of speech, types of sentences (declarative, interrogative, passive, etc.)
      2. Noun phrase/verb phrase, phrase structure tree
      3. Deep structure, syntactic ambiguity
   D. Pragmatics
      1. Communicative intentions and speech acts
      2. Stages of pragmatic development
      3. Narratives and conversational rules

Praxis Area 2: Assessment and Diagnosis

I. **Phonology and Speech Sound Disorders**
   A. Recognize and classify speech sound disorders according to phonological features
   B. Relate speech sound disorders to anatomical and physiological etiology
   C. Differentiate functional and organic disorders

II. **Semantic and Syntactical Language Disorders**
   A. Identify abnormal development, receptive, and expressive disorders
   B. Calculate Mean Length of Utterance (MLU) and type/token ratio and relate to severity of language delay
   C. Identify semantic and syntactic characteristics of adult neurological disorders
   D. Collect and analyze language samples
   E. Identify and classify syntactical errors
   F. Relate syntactical errors to etiology, type, and severity of disorders

III. **Pragmatic Language Disorders**
   A. Relate pragmatic development to identification of disorders in early childhood
   B. Relate pragmatic language behavior to autism spectrum disorder and traumatic brain injury
   C. Identify language learning disability and pragmatic language disorder

Praxis Area 3: Treatment Planning and Evaluation

I. Articulation, Language, and Motor Speech Disorders
   A. Select treatment targets and response classes based on structural complexity and cultural appropriateness
   B. Formulate long-term goals and short-term objectives based on assessment outcomes and developmental sequence
   C. Evaluate performance outcomes based on normal linguistic behavior

Sample Linguistics Question

When spoken aloud, the sentence "She's a good cook your mother" is comprehensible because:

   A. It is accurate according to grammatical rules

   B. Its deep structure meaning is implied

   C. It is structurally unambiguous

   D. It is a dialectal construction

If you are uncertain of the answer, the reasoning process of critiquing can be used to eliminate options. Using critiquing, (A), (C), and (D) should be eliminated since the sentence is ungrammatical, ambiguous, and not typical of any dialect. In syntactic analysis, surface structure refers to the arrangement of words according to grammatical rules, as in "Your mother, [she] is a good cook." However, deep structure rules allow rearrangement of phrase constituents to convey the same meaning. Although the sentence is ungrammatical, it is nonetheless comprehensible, and (B) is correct.

Suggested Linguistics Study Resources

Fromkin, V., Rodman, R., & Hyams, N. (2019). *An introduction to language.* Independence, KY: Cengage.

Singleton, N., & Shulman, B. (2015). Language acquisition: Preverbal and early language. In G. Lof & A. Johnson (Eds.), *National speech-language pathology examination review and study guide* (pp. 79–90). Evanston, IL: TherapyEd.

Roseberry-McKibbin, C., & Hegde, M. (2018). Language development in children. In *Advanced review of speech-language pathology* (pp. 105–146). Austin, TX: Pro-Ed.

Language Development

Praxis Area 1: Foundations

I. Terminology and Concepts

Behaviorist theory, Bootstrapping, Brown's stages, Communicative intent, Concrete operations, Copula, Developmental milestones, Fast mapping, Formal operations, Holophrastic stage, Illocutionary, Imbedded clause, Indirect speech act, Joint reference, Language Acquisition Device (LAD), Lexicon, Locutionary, Mand, Narrative, Nativist theory, Overgeneralization, Perlocutionary, Preoperational stage, Reduplication, Referent, Scaffolding, Self-correction, Semantic relation, Sensorimotor stage, Speech act, Surface structure, Tact, Telegraphic speech

II. **Stages and Sequence of Emergence of Linguistic Elements by Age Level**
   A. Pragmatic Development
      1. Perlocutionary, illocutionary, and locutionary stages
      2. Preverbal communicative intentions
   B. Phonological Development
      1. Emergence and suppression of phonological processes
   C. Semantic Development
      1. Holophrastic stage, two-word construction of meaning
      2. Semantic relations, function words
      3. Word learning
   D. Morphological Development
      1. Brown's stages (MLU)
      2. Mastery levels
      3. Indicators of language disorder
   E. Syntactic Development
      1. Expansion of MLU
      2. Expansion of sentence types and complexity
      3. Sentence comprehension skills
      4. Emergence of literacy

III. **Theories of Language Acquisition**
   A. Piaget's stages of cognitive development
   B. Skinner's behaviorist theory/Nativist theory
   C. Language Acquisition Device (LAD)
   D. Caregiver facilitation and influence of environment
   E. Joint reference, bootstrapping, scaffolding, input deprivation
   F. Bilingual language learning

Praxis Area 2: Assessment and Diagnosis

I. **Determination of Language Disorders**
   A. Identify language delay, receptive and expressive disorders
   B. Relate error frequency and form to etiology, type, and severity of disorders
   C. Calculate MLU and type/token ratio and relate to severity level
   D. Collect and analyze language samples

Praxis Area 3: Treatment Planning and Evaluation

I. Intervention for Language Disorders
   A. Determine treatment targets for type and severity of disorder
   B. Utilize developmental sequence in formulation of goals and objectives
   C. Determine treatment strategies based on learning theories
   D. Select appropriate stimuli and performance tasks to facilitate language learning

Sample Language Development Question

A 5-year-old girl makes substitution errors involving the phonemes /r/, /l/, tʃ/, and /s/. Her auditory comprehension age is 4.0 years, and she has a verbal ability age of approximately 2.5 years. Her expressive language is typified by utterances of one to three words in length with no morphological inflections. Findings on measures of hearing and emotional status are negative. On the basis of this information, the speech-language-pathologist could most appropriately begin to:[1]

   A. Correct production of /r/ and /s/ in all positions and help the child achieve carryover into spontaneous speech

   B. Teach recognition and naming of primary colors and develop production of plural allomorphs /-s/ and /-z/

   C. Teach discrimination of /s/ in isolation and in syllables and work on correct production of /s/ in initial positions

   D. Increase expressive vocabulary and work on present progressive tense (noun + "-ing" verb constructions)

Clinical decision-making questions such as this require the reasoning skills of comparison and classification, which are performed on the answer choices by comparing each to the other and placing them in hierarchical status. In addition, application of your knowledge of language acquisition is important. Since the child's verbal ability lags behind her auditory comprehension age, and since both lag behind her chronological age, at this stage, the primary goal should be to expand language skills. Hence, work on articulation and plural allomorphs are less important, so (A), (B), and (C) are incorrect. Following the sequence of language development, treatment should focus on increasing vocabulary and mean length of utterance (MLU) beginning with present progressive tense "-ing" since these are early morphological forms. Therefore, (D) is the correct answer. Note that each answer choice is a compound statement containing two possible actions. The correct answer must reflect the statement where both actions are viable.

Suggested Language Development Study Resources

Owens, R. (2016). *Language development: An introduction.* Boston, MA: Pearson.
Singleton, N., & Shulman, B. (2015). Language acquisition: Preverbal and early language. In G. Lof & A. Johnson (Eds.), *National speech-language pathology examination review and study guide.* (pp. 79–90). Evanston, IL: TherapyEd.

Lof, G., & Watson, M. (2015). Speech sound disorders in children. In G. Lof & A. Johnson (Eds.), *National speech-language pathology examination review and study guide.* (pp. 139–166). Evanston, IL: TherapyEd.

Roseberry-McKibbin, C., & Hegde, M. (2018). Language development in children. In *Advanced review of speech-language pathology.* Austin, TX: Pro-Ed.

Roseberry-McKibbin, C., & Hegde, M. (2018). Articulatory-phonological development and speech sound disorders. In *Advanced review of speech-language pathology.* (pp. 207–252). Austin, TX: Pro-Ed.

Phonetics

Praxis Area 1: Foundations

I. **Terminology and Concepts**
Accent, Affricate, Allophone, Alveolar, Anterior sound, Aspiration, Back vowel, Central vowel, Cluster, Cognate, Continuant, Coronal, Dialect, Diphthong, Distinctive features, Dorsal, Epenthesis, Formant, Free variation, Fricative, Front vowels, Glide, High/Mid/Low vowels, Interdental, International Phonetic Alphabet (IPA), Intonation, Labial, Labiodental, Lateral, Lax, Lingual, Liquid, Minimal pair, Nasal, Obstruent, Palatal, Palatoalveolar, Prosody, Resonance, Sibilant, Sonorant, Standard English, Stop, Strident, Suprasegmental, Syllable structure (Consonant-Vowel [CV]; Consonant-Vowel-Consonant [CVC])]), Tense vowel, Voiced/Unvoiced-Voiceless sound, Velar

II. **Phoneme Classification**
   A. Voicing, manner, and place of articulation
   B. Vowel height, placement, and tension
   C. Acoustical characteristics of consonants and vowels/formants
   D. Distinctive feature identification and analysis

III. **Phonetic Transcription**
   A. IPA representations
   B. Broad and narrow transcription notations

Praxis Area 2: Assessment and Diagnosis

I. **Administration and Interpretation of Articulation Tests**
   A. Transcribe spoken sounds
   B. Distinguish normal phoneme production from errors
   C. Classify errors according to phonetic features (substitutions, omissions, deletions, additions)
   D. Classify errors according to phonemic characteristics (place, manner, voicing, acoustics, distinctive features)

  E. Identify potential effects on articulation from oral examination, and organic and structural deficiencies

II. **Determination of Speech Sound Disorders**
  A. Relate errors to organic, structural, and functional etiology
  B. Classify degree of severity of disorders

Praxis Area 3: Treatment Planning and Evaluation

 I. **Intervention for Articulation and Motor Speech Disorders**
  A. Determine treatment targets and strategies appropriate for the type of disorder
  B. Formulate long-term goals, short-term objectives, and targets for intervention
  C. Describe and document progress and outcomes

Sample Phonetics Question

Production of "tests" as [tɛsɪz] by a client with Broca aphasia who speaks a variety of African-American English illustrates which of the following?[2]

  A. Apraxia of speech

  B. Dialectally appropriate formation

  C. Dysarthria

  D. Phonemic paraphasia

Assuming that you recognize that the client's pronunciation of [tɛstz] is phonetically transcribed as /tɛs/ + /ɪz/, where the difference is reflected in the final plural morpheme, it should be evident that the question requires the reasoning skill of critiquing. Critiquing each option in sequence, (A) should be eliminated since apraxia is most likely to affect the initial phoneme. Similarly, (C) and (D) should be eliminated since there is no phonemic error in the client's pronunciation. The correct answer is (B) since speakers of African-American English often formulate plurality in words ending in a consonant cluster by reducing the cluster and applying the regular plural, hence [tɛstz] is realized as [tɛsɪz]. The question might also be answered by cluing, since the client's ethnicity is identified in the question, and answer choice (B) hints of nonbiased assessment procedures.

Suggested Phonetics Study Resources

Small, L. (2016). *Fundamentals of phonetics.* Boston, MA: Pearson.

Singleton, N., & Shulman, B. (2015). Language acquisition: Preverbal and early language. In G. Lof & A. Johnson (Eds.), *National speech-language pathology examination review and study guide.* (pp. 79–90). Evanston, IL: TherapyEd.

Roseberry-McKibbin, C., & Hegde, M. (2018). Physiological and acoustic phonetics. In *Advanced review of speech-language pathology.* (pp. 69–102). Austin, TX: Pro-Ed.

Anatomy and Physiology

Praxis Area 1: Foundations

I. **Terminology and Concepts**
Abdominal muscles, Abduct/Adduct, Alveolar ridge, Articulators, Arytenoid muscle/cartilage, Cranial nerve innervations, Cricoid cartilage/bone, Diaphragm, Epiglottis, Facial muscles, Hard palate, Hyoid cartilage/bone, Incus, Inner ear, Intercostal muscles, Intrinsic/Extrinsic laryngeal muscles, Intrinsic/Extrinsic tongue muscles, Larynx, Malleus, Mandible, Middle ear, Muscles of inspiration/expiration, Nasal cavity, Oral cavity, Palatal muscles, Pharynx, Soft palate, Stapes, Thyroid bone, Trachea, True/False vocal folds, Tympanic membrane, Velum

II. **Normal Hearing and Speech Production**
   A. Breathing, voice production, articulation, and hearing
      1. Identify and locate muscles, bones, and cartilages
      2. Describe normal functions of muscles, bones, and cartilages

Praxis Area 2: Assessment and Diagnosis

I. **Assessment of Structural Impairment on Speech and Hearing**
   A. Recognize symptoms, disease conditions, orofacial anomalies, and syndromes
   B. Identify and predict speech and hearing manifestations of physical impairment
   C. Identify locus of physical impairment based on speech and hearing characteristics

II. **Instrumentation and Testing Procedures**
   A. Assess extent of impairment
   B. Conduct differential diagnosis (especially motor speech disorders)
   C. Classify degree of severity of speech and hearing disorders
   D. Conduct hearing screening
   E. Provide prognosis for recovery

Praxis Area 3: Treatment Planning and Evaluation

I. **Utilization of Diagnostic Information for Intervention**
   A. Identify appropriate treatment approaches
   B. Construct realistic and relevant goals and objectives based on type and severity of disorder
   C. Implement relevant treatment procedures
   D. Evaluate and document treatment outcomes
   E. Make appropriate referrals

Sample Anatomy and Physiology Question

Which of the following best describes the most common deficit, if any, caused solely by an unusually high but intact palatal vault?[3]

    A. There is no typical speech deficit.

    B. High front vowels cannot be distinguished from high back vowels.

    C. Most palatal consonants are produced incorrectly.

    D. Nasal consonants cannot be distinguished from their oral counterparts.

Abstract reasoning and comparison are reasoning skills that will assist in answering the question. Use abstract reasoning to determine the impact of a high palatal vault on speech. Use comparison to rule out untenable answer choices. Taken alone, palatal vault height does not have a significant impact on speech production since tongue and velar movement compensate to produce speech, so (B), (C), and (D) should be eliminated. Furthermore, use comparison to eliminate (B) and (C) since high front and back vowels, as well as palatal consonants, result from tongue placement rather than palatal vault height. Similarly, (D) should be eliminated because nasal consonants are distinguished from oral consonants by nasal emission rather than palatal vault height. Therefore (A) is the correct answer. A clue to confirm the correct answer is found in the statement "if any" in the question.

Suggested Anatomy and Physiology Study Resources

Kent, R., & Vorperian, H. (2011). The biology and physics of speech. In N. Anderson & G. Shames (Eds.), *Human communication disorders: An introduction*. Boston, MA: Pearson.

Heaton, J., & Vallila-Rohter, S. (2015). Anatomy and physiology of communication and swallowing. In G. Lof & A. Johnson (Eds.), *National speech-language pathology examination review and study guide* (pp. 1–46). Evanston, IL: TherapyEd.

Roseberry-McKibbin, C., & Hegde, M. (2018). Anatomy, neuroanatomy and physiology of the speech mechanism. In *Advanced review of speech-language pathology* (pp. 1–15). Austin, TX: Pro-Ed.

Diagnostic Methods

Praxis Area 1: Foundations

  I. Terminology and Concepts

      Age equivalency, Age range, Authentic assessment, Baseline, Candidacy for AAC device, Case history, Causality, Cognitive tests, Counseling, Criterion referenced test, Diagnostic report, Differential diagnosis (especially neurogenic language and motor speech disorders), Dynamic assessment, Ethnographic interview, Etiology, Functional assessment, Instrumentation (voice/swallowing), IEP goal/

team, Interview protocol, Language sample/analysis, Naturalistic observation, Norming sample, Norm referenced test, Orofacial examination, Percentile, Portfolio assessment, Prognostic indicators, Raw score, Recommendations, Reliability, Screening, Severity, Standardized test, Standard score, Stanine, Testing procedures, Test interpretation, Test limitations, Test selection, Validity

Praxis Area 2: Assessment and Diagnosis

I. **Principles of Diagnosis**
   A. Identify purpose for various assessments
   B. Recognize and identify etiologic factors of speech and language disorders

II. **Administration, Scoring, and Interpretation of Assessment Instruments**
   A. Select appropriate tests/instruments and interpret results
   B. Identify and classify severity of a disorder by speech and language characteristics
   C. Distinguish normal development and behaviors from errors and disorders
   D. Identify elements of the assessment battery and diagnostic report
   E. Recognize and classify prognostic indicators; formulate a prognosis
   F. Recognize defense mechanisms and need for counseling

Praxis Area 3: Treatment Planning and Evaluation

I. **Treatment Principles**
   A. Make appropriate referrals for additional tests and treatment
   B. Relate diagnosis to specific treatment program or approach to treatment

II. **Implementation of Treatment Procedures**
   A. Utilize baseline data for measuring and tracking treatment progress
   B. Select target behaviors for intervention based on assessment outcomes
   C. Plan sequential treatment goals and objectives based on type, severity, and nature of speech and language characteristics
   D. Identify and distinguish treatment methods and recognize the treatment most likely to promote success

Sample Diagnostic Methods Question

During a kindergarten screening, a 5-year-old child who has never had speech-language services is judged to misarticulate the /s/ and /r/ sounds. Which of the following factors is predictive of the child's ability to improve articulatory /s/ and /r/ skills on a developmental basis without intervention?[4]

   A. The rate of repeating [p ə t ə k ə] on a diadochokinetic task
   B. High score on a general test of auditory discrimination ability

C. Good general verbal aptitude

D. Correct production of target sounds in response to stimulation by the clinician

The reasoning skill of critiquing should be used to compare each answer choice to the specifications of the question. The question relates to spontaneous emergence of /s/ and /r/, which are later-developing sounds. Using comparison, choices (A), (B), and (C) should be eliminated since they do not directly relate to spontaneous phonological development, although they may be causes for a disorder in an older child. Thus, the correct answer is (D), which relates to stimulability of the target sounds, which is the best predictor of spontaneous emergence.

Suggested Diagnostic Methods Study Resources

Shipley, K., & McAfee, J. (2019). *Assessment in speech-language pathology: A resource manual.* San Diego, CA: Plural Publishing.

Greenwald, M. (2015). Research, evidence-based practice and tests and measurements. In G. Lof & A. Johnson (Eds.), *National speech-language pathology examination review and study guide.* Evanston, IL: TherapyEd.

Roseberry-McKibbin, C., & Hegde, M. (2018). Assessment and treatment: Principles of evidence-based practice. In *Advanced review of speech-language pathology* (pp. 515–562). Austin, TX: Pro-Ed.

Roseberry-McKibbin, C., & Hegde, M. (2018). Special topics in speech-language pathology—Counseling. In *Advanced review of speech-language pathology* (pp. 601–646). Austin, TX: Pro-Ed.

Clinical Methods

Praxis Area 1: Foundations

I. **Terminology and Concepts**

Antecedent, Applied behavior analysis, ASHA Code of Ethics, Aversive stimulus, Behavior modification, Caseload, Cloze procedure, Contingency, Continuous reinforcement, Counseling, Criterion, Early intervention, Expansion, Extension, Extinction, Fading, Follow-up, Generalization, Goal, IEP goal/objective, Maintenance, Mand-tact, Mastery, Modeling, Negative reinforcement, Operant conditioning, Outcome measures, Probe, Prompt, Punishment, Referral, Reinforcement schedule/Reinforcer, Response class, Response cost, Response shaping, Response to Intervention (RTI), Reward, Subjective-Objective-Assessment-Plan (SOAP) note, Speech-Language Pathology Scope of Practice, Stimulus, Target behavior, Token economy, Tracking progress, Treatment continuum/sequence, Treatment planning, Treatment termination

Praxis Area 2: Assessment and Diagnosis

I. Utilization of Diagnostic Information for Planning Intervention
   A. Record and analyze performance data to evaluate and document progress
   B. Identify and prioritize target behaviors for intervention
   C. Recommend frequency of intervention
   D. Identify need for referral

Praxis Area 3: Treatment Planning and Evaluation

I. Planning and Implementation of Treatment Procedures
   A. Identify purpose and functions of treatment approaches and procedures
   B. Identify the treatment method most likely to promote success
   C. Recognize elements of, and construct, a behavioral objective
   D. Determine most effective strategy to elicit and maintain desired behavior
   E. Prioritize steps in the treatment process
   F. Manage extraneous behaviors that interfere with treatment
   G. Recognize client counseling approaches and techniques

II. Evaluation of Performance and Outcomes
   A. Utilize performance data to document progress
   B. Utilize performance data to determine next step or terminate treatment
   C. Recognize examples of unethical behavior

Sample Clinical Methods Question

When rhythm or metronome-paced intervention is used for clients who stutter, weekly clinical intervention sessions should be terminated and replaced by monthly maintenance sessions when the client has met which of the following criteria?[5]

   A. Thirty minutes of the client's spontaneous conversational speech in the clinical setting contains between 10 and 15 dysfluencies.

   B. The client has attended weekly group meetings for several months to practice relaxation, self-evaluation, simulation rehearsal, and desensitization.

   C. The client has practiced conversational exchange in five settings outside the clinic and self-reported an 85 percent reduction rate in dysfluencies over a period of 3 months.

   D. In conversations held outside the clinical sessions, the client reports experiencing decreased anxiety, tension, and stress.

Selection of the correct answer should involve the reasoning skills of classification, predicting the examiner, and values. Using classification, you should eliminate answers by examining each and placing them in hierarchical order. The correct answer should be the most thorough and efficacious action. Therefore, (A), (B), and (D) should be eliminated since they are incomplete. Furthermore, using predicting the examiner and values, you should recognize the correct answer as (C) because it is most thorough in terms of data collection and it represents the values of the profession.

Suggested Clinical Methods Study Resources

Greenwald, M. (2015). Research, evidence-based practice and tests and measurements. In G. Lof & A. Johnson (Eds.), *National speech-language pathology examination review and study guide* (pp. 91–102). Evanston, IL: TherapyEd.

Roseberry-McKibbin, C., & Hegde, M. (2018). Assessment and treatment: Principles of evidence-based practice. In *Advanced review of speech-language pathology* (pp. 515–562). Austin, TX: Pro-Ed.

Roseberry-McKibbin, C., & Hegde, M. (2018). Special topics in speech-language pathology— Counseling. In *Advanced review of speech-language pathology* (pp. 601–666). Austin, TX: Pro-Ed.

Audiology

Praxis Area 1: Foundations

I. Terminology and Concepts

Air-bone gap, Air conduction, Assistive listening device, Audiogram, Auditory-verbal approach, Aural rehabilitation, Bilateral/Unilateral loss, Bone conduction, Cochlear implant, Conductive/Sensorineural/Mixed loss, Counseling, Deaf, Deaf culture, Incus, Malleus, Masking, Meniere's disease, Mild/Moderate/Severe/Profound loss, Oral/Aural approach, Otitis media, Otosclerosis, Otoscopic examination, Phonetically balanced (PB) word list, Presbycusis, Pure-tone audiometry, Pure-tone average, Screening frequencies/level, Speech banana, Speech-Language Pathology Scope of Practice, Speech recognition threshold, Spondee word list, Tinnitus, Tympanogram

Praxis Area 2: Assessment and Diagnosis

I. Effects of Hearing Loss on Speech and Language Disorders
   A. Conduct a pure-tone hearing screening
   B. Read and interpret an audiogram
   C. Recognize type and level of hearing loss
   D. Predict effect of hearing level on receptive and expressive speech and language development

Praxis Area 3: Treatment Planning and Evaluation

I. Speech and Language Intervention for Hearing Loss
   A. Make appropriate referrals

    B. Conduct aural rehabilitation procedures

    C. Conduct speech training for individuals with cochlear implants

Sample Audiology Question

Which of the following would be indicative of an air-bone gap?[6]

    A. Air conduction thresholds 10 dB worse than bone conduction thresholds from 250 to 4000 Hz

    B. A Carhart notch

    C. Reduced sensitivity to frequencies above 4000 Hz

    D. Bone conduction thresholds 10 dB worse than air conduction thresholds from 250 to 4000 Hz

This is an example of a verbatim recall question. If you decided to eliminate (A) and (D), perhaps you were tempted to use the test-taking strategy of avoiding opposites, but using cluing as a reasoning skill would be a better choice because the question contains the word *gap* and neither a Carhart notch or reduced frequencies above 4000 Hz suggests a gap. Recall from your study that bone conduction is generally better than air conduction. This knowledge should lead you to the correct choice, which is (A).

Suggested Audiology Study Resources

Martin, F., & Noble, B. (2011). Hearing and hearing disorders. In N. Anderson & G. Shames (Eds.), *Human communication disorders: An introduction* (pp. 504–537). Boston, MA: Pearson.

Holmes, A., & Thomas, N. (2011). Audiologic rehabilitation. In N. Anderson & G. Shames (Eds.), *Human communication disorders: An introduction* (pp. 538–564). Boston, MA: Pearson.

Newman, C., Sandridge, S., & Goldberg, D. (2015). Audiology and hearing impairment. In G. Lof & A. Johnson (Eds.), *National speech-language pathology examination review and study guide* (pp. 409–438). Evanston: IL: TherapyEd.

Roseberry-McKibbin, C., & Hegde, M. (2018). Audiology and hearing disorders. In *Advanced review of speech-language pathology* (pp. 463–514). Austin, TX: Pro-Ed.

Roseberry-McKibbin, C., & Hegde, M. (2018). Special topics in speech-language pathology—Counseling. In *Advanced review of speech-language pathology* (pp. 601–607). Austin, TX: Pro-Ed.

Neuroanatomy/Neurophysiology

Praxis Area 1: Foundations

    I. Terminology and Concepts

Brain stem, Broca's area, Carotid artery, Central nervous system, Cerebellum, Cerebrovascular accident (CVA), Circle of Willis, Corpus collosum, Cranial nerves, Decussation, Frontal lobe, Glial cell, Middle cerebral artery, Motor cortex, Myelin, Occipital lobe, Parietal lobe, Peripheral nervous system, Pons, Pyramidal/Extrapyramidal system, Sensory/Motor neuron, Spinal nerve, Soma, Temporal lobe, Upper/Lower motor neuron, Wernicke's area

II. **Normal Language Development and Comprehension**
   A. Identify and label structures and areas of the brain with relation to receptive and expressive speech and language
   B. Describe normal brain function for speech and language

Praxis Area 2: Assessment and Diagnosis

I. **Effects of Structural Impairments on Speech and Language**
   A. Identify and predict speech and language manifestations of damage or impairment
   B. Identify locus of impairment based on speech and hearing characteristics
   C. Identify, distinguish, and label medical conditions based on symptoms

II. **Instrumentation and Testing Procedures**
   A. Assess extent of speech and language impairment
   B. Conduct differential diagnosis of motor speech disorders and neurogenic language disorders
   C. Classify degree of severity of speech and language disorders
   D. Formulate prognosis for recovery

Praxis Area 3: Treatment Planning and Evaluation

I. **Utilization of Diagnostic Information for Intervention**
   A. Identify appropriate treatment approaches
   B. Construct realistic and relevant goals and objectives
   C. Implement systematic treatment procedures
   D. Evaluate and document treatment outcomes

Sample Neuroanatomy/Neurophysiology Question

Which of the following disorders is most likely to accompany a marked aphasia resulting from a single left-hemisphere cerebrovascular accident?[7]

   A. Apraxia of speech
   B. Spastic dysarthria
   C. Left hemiparesis
   D. Prosopagnosia

Although they often require verbatim recall, neuroanatomy and neurophysiology questions are generally presented in an applied clinical context such as this question where critiquing is the reasoning skill that should be used. Spastic dysarthria is a motor speech disorder usually arising from bilateral lesions, so (B) should be eliminated. Left hemiparesis is caused by a right hemisphere CVA, so (C) is also incorrect. If you are not familiar with prosopagnosia, you should exercise a test-taking strategy and not select unfamiliar terms, leaving (A), which is the correct answer since apraxia of speech often accompanies aphasia.

Suggested Neuroanatomy/ Neurophysiology Study Resources

Nicholas, M. (2015). Acquired language disorders: Aphasia, right-hemisphere disorders and neurogenerative syndromes. In G. Lof & A. Johnson (Eds.), *National speech-language pathology examination review and study guide* (pp. 255–298). Evanston, IL: TherapyEd.

Roseberry-McKibbin, C., & Hegde, M. (2018). Neuroanatomy and neurophysiology: The nervous system. In *Advanced review of speech-language pathology* (pp. 28–67). Austin, TX: Pro-Ed.

Articulation Disorders

Praxis Area 1: Foundations

I. Terminology and Concepts
Addition, Ankyloglossia, Apraxia, Cleft lip/palate, Contrastive analysis, Craniofacial anomalies, Cycles approach, Developmental apraxia, Diadochokinesis, Distinctive feature analysis/approach, Distortion, Dysarthria, Ear training, Functional disorder, Generalization, Genetic syndromes, Intelligibility, Malocclusion, Multiple phoneme approach, Omission, Orofacial syndromes, Paired stimuli approach, Phonemic awareness, Phonological process/analysis, Place-Manner-Voicing, Prosody, Sensorimotor approach, Stimulability, Substitution, Successive approximations, Tongue thrust

II. Phonetics, Phonology, and Normal Speech Production
   A. IPA symbols, distinctive features, Place-Manner-Voicing
   B. Anatomy and physiology of speech

Praxis Area 2: Assessment and Diagnosis

I. Implementation of Assessment Procedures
   A. Recognize and classify type and severity of disorders

    B. Identify and distinguish characteristics and functions of articulation tests

    C. Select appropriate tests based on purpose and age range

    D. Conduct orofacial examination; describe effects on speech production

II. **Interpretation of Assessment Results**

    A. Identify and transcribe error sounds

    B. Relate disorders to anatomical and physiological etiology

    C. Differentiate functional and organic disorders

    D. Differentiate articulation disorders from dialect and second language influences

Praxis Area 3: Treatment Planning and Evaluation

I. **Utilization of Diagnostic Information for Planning Intervention**

    A. Apply developmental milestones and phonological process analysis in formulation of goals and objectives

    B. Select appropriate intervention approach, elicitation techniques, materials, and performance tasks

II. **Implementation of Treatment Procedures**

    A. Determine treatment targets based on type and severity of disorder

    B. Implement specific approaches and treatment programs

    C. Prioritize steps in the treatment process

    D. Utilize outcome data to determine next step or terminate treatment

Sample Articulation Disorders Question

A 4-year-old child whose speech is 70% unintelligible and who has normal neuro-muscular functioning is referred for an assessment. Which of the following evaluation methods would be most useful in planning intervention?[8]

    A. Preschool Language Scale

    B. Fisher-Logeman Test of Articulation

    C. MacDonald Deep Test of Articulation

    D. Khan-Lewis Phonological Process Analysis

Cluing would be a useful reasoning skill since the question specifies that the child has normal neuromuscular functioning. Thus, the correct answer should relate to functional assessment, which would be accomplished by the Khan-Lewis Phonological Process Analysis, or (D). (A) should be eliminated since the Preschool Language Scale is not strictly an articulation test. The MacDonald Deep Test is unlikely to yield information on phonological processes, so (C) should be eliminated. Since the Khan-Lewis test uses data from the Goldman-Fristoe test, (B) should be eliminated.

Suggested Articulation Disorders Study Resources

Schwartz, R., & Marton, K. (2011). Articulatory and phonological disorders. In N. Anderson & G. Shames (Eds.), *Human communication disorders: An introduction* (pp. 149–182). Boston, MA: Pearson.

Lof, G., & Watson, M. (2015). Speech sound disorders in children. In G. Lof & A. Johnson (Eds.), *National speech-language pathology examination review and study guide* (pp. 139–166). Evanston, IL: TherapyEd.

Roseberry-McKibbin, C., & Hegde, M. (2018). Articulatory-phonological development and speech sound disorders. In *Advanced review of speech-language pathology* (pp. 207–252). Austin, TX: Pro-Ed.

Language Disorders

Praxis Area 1: Foundations

I. **Terminology and Concepts**
Attention Deficit Hyperactivity Disorder (ADHD), Authentic assessment, Autism spectrum disorder, Cerebral palsy, Cloze, Criterion referenced test, Dynamic assessment, Expansion, Expressive/Receptive disorder, Extension, Fading, Interdisciplinary Family Service Plan/Individualized Education Plan (IFSP/IEP), Imitation, Incidental teaching, Intellectual disability, Joint routines, Language age, Language disorder/delay, Language learning disability, Language sampling techniques/analysis, Mand-model, Mean length of utterance (MLU), Milieu teaching, Modeling, Parallel talk, Physical/Social/Environmental risk factors, Portfolio assessment, Prompting, Reauditorization, Recasting, Response to Intervention (RTI), Self-talk, Semantic/Syntactic/Morphological/Pragmatic disorder characteristics, Shaping, Specific language impairment, Stanine, Type/Token ratio, Whole language approach

Praxis Area 2: Assessment and Diagnosis

I. **Implementation of Assessment Procedures**
   A. Identify alternatives to standardized tests
   B. Collect and analyze language samples
   C. Calculate MLU and type/token ratio and relate to severity level

II. **Interpretation of Assessment Results**
   A. Distinguish normal developmental characteristics from errors
   B. Identify and distinguish language delay, receptive and expressive disorders
   C. Identify and classify language tests according to purpose, scope, and age range
   D. Select, administer, and interpret results of language tests
   E. Relate errors and frequency to etiology, type, and severity of disorders

    F. Relate disorder characteristics to other developmental and cognitive disabilities

Praxis Area 3: Treatment Planning and Evaluation

  I. **Utilization of Diagnostic Information for Planning Intervention**
    A. Use developmental sequence to plan treatment, select and prioritize target behaviors
    B. Utilize test results to select treatment approaches and programs and prioritize target behaviors

 II. **Implementation of Treatment Procedures**
    A. Identify and label treatment approaches and programs
    B. Identify the treatment method most likely to promote success
    C. Determine most effective strategy to elicit and maintain desired behavior
    D. Prioritize steps in the treatment process
    E. Apply normal acquisition processes as techniques for eliciting target behaviors
    F. Utilize performance data to determine next step, alter or terminate treatment
    G. Manage extraneous behaviors that interfere with treatment
    H. Work collaboratively with other professionals

Sample Language Disorders Question

A speech-language pathologist using the modeling technique to stimulate expressive language skills in a child typically does which of the following?[9]
    A. Repeats what the child says without adding to the utterance
    B. Repeats what the child says, then adds to the utterance, explaining the child's errors
    C. Uses gestures along with words whenever there is communication with the child
    D. Provides an example for the child to repeat

Both critiquing and comparison should be applied to this question. First, using critiquing, (A) and (C) should be eliminated since both are unlikely to stimulate the child's speech production. Using comparison with (B) and (D), (C) should be eliminated since there is no expectation for the child to speak. Thus, (B) is the correct answer.

Suggested Language Disorders Study Resources

Bacon, C., & Wilcox, J. (2011). Developmental language impairment in infancy and early childhood. In N. Anderson & G. Shames (Eds.), *Human communication disorders: An introduction* (pp. 325–351). Boston, MA: Pearson.

Culatta, B., & Wiig, E. (2011). Language disabilities in school-age children and youth. In N. Anderson & G. Shames (Eds.), *Human communication disorders: An introduction* (pp. 352–385). Boston, MA: Pearson.

Weiss, A. (2015). Language disorders in young children. In G. Lof & A. Johnson (Eds.), *National speech-language pathology examination review and study guide* (pp. 167–192). Evanston, IL: TherapyEd.

Guillam, S., & Simonsmeier, V. (2015). Spoken language disorders in school-age populations. In G. Lof & A. Johnson (Eds.), *National speech-language pathology examination review and study guide* (pp. 198–208). Evanston, IL: TherapyEd.

Richard, G. (2015). Autism spectrum disorders. In G. Lof & A. Johnson (Eds.), *National speech-language pathology examination review and study guide* (pp. 225–240). Evanston, IL: TherapyEd.

Roseberry-McKibbin, C., & Hegde, M. (2018). Language disorders in children. In *Advanced review of speech-language pathology* (pp. 149–206). Austin, TX: Pro-Ed.

Stuttering

Praxis Area 1: Foundations

I. **Terminology and Concepts**
   Adaptation effect, Airflow, Avoidance, Blending, Blocks, Broken words, Circumlocution, Cluttering, Consistency effect, Counseling, Delayed auditory feedback, Desensitization, Diagnosogenic-Semantogenic Theory, Easy onset, Environmental manipulation, Fluency reinforcement, Fluency shaping, Incomplete sentences, Interjections, Neurogenic stuttering, Normal dysfluency, Operant behavior theory, Parent-directed intervention, Prolongation, Prolonged speech, Psychoneuroses, Rate reduction, Repetition, Revision, Rhythmic speech, Secondary behavior, Soft contact, Time-out

Praxis Area 2: Assessment and Diagnosis

I. **Principles of Stuttering Assessment**
   A. Identify and administer fluency assessment instruments and protocols
   B. Recognize adaptation/consistency effects
   C. Classify stuttering severity

II. **Implementation of Assessment Protocols and Interpret Results**
   A. Identify and distinguish theories of stuttering etiology
   B. Distinguish normal dysfluency from stuttering in preschool children
   C. Identify, label, and describe behavioral and psychological characteristics of stuttering

Praxis Area 3: Treatment Planning and Evaluation

I. Principles of Treatment
   A. Identify and describe treatment approaches and techniques
   B. Relate theories of etiology to treatment approaches
   C. Recognize purpose and goals for various treatment techniques

II. Implementation of Treatment Procedures
   A. Identify the treatment method most likely to promote success
   B. Implement procedures to promote and sustain fluency
   C. Collect and utilize performance data to evaluate performance outcomes
   D. Identify need for and techniques of counseling

Sample Stuttering Question

When successful, fluency shaping techniques for a client who stutters accomplish which of the following?[10]

   A. Lessen the client's ability to generalize fluent speech in new situations

   B. Reduce the frequency of stuttering but require the client to pay attention to the act of talking

   C. Reduce the number of speech situations that the client attempts

   D. Lessen the duration of stuttering behaviors but not the frequency with which they occur

You should immediately recognize a clue in the question, which is the phrase "when successful." This means that (A) and (C) should be eliminated since they are not desirable outcomes of stuttering treatment. Similarly, using critiquing to decide between (B) and (D), (D) should be eliminated since a treatment strategy that does not reduce the frequency of stuttering would not be successful. Therefore, (B) is the correct answer.

Suggested Stuttering Study Resources

Ramig, P., & Pollard, R. (2011). Stuttering and other disorders of fluency. In N. Anderson & G. Shames (Eds.), *Human communication disorders: An introduction* (pp. 183–221). Boston, MA: Pearson.

Daniels, D., & Johnson, A. (2015). Stuttering and other fluency disorders. In G. Lof & A. Johnson (Eds.), *National speech-language pathology examination review and study guide* (pp. 241–254). Evanston, IL: TherapyEd.

Roseberry-McKibbin, C., & Hegde, M. (2018). Fluency and its disorders. In *Advanced review of speech-language pathology* (pp. 253–289). Austin, TX: Pro-Ed.

Voice Disorders

Praxis Area 1: Foundations

I. Terminology and Concepts
Alaryngeal/Esophageal speech, Ankylosis, Arytenoids, Blom-Sanger device, Breathiness, Clavicular breathing, Contact ulcer, Conversion aphonia, Cul-de-sac, Diplophonia, Electrolarynx, Electromyography, Endoscopy, Fundamental frequency, Glottal fry, Granuloma, Harshness, Hemangioma, Hoarseness, Hyper/Hyponasality, Injection/Inhalation device, Laryngectomy, Laryngoscopy, Maximal phonation time, Nasometer, Papilloma, Pharyngeal-esophageal segment (PES), Pitch, Pitch breaks, s/z ratio, Spasmodic dysphonia, Stoma, Strain-strangle, Strident, Teflon treatment, Videostrobsoscopy, Visi-pitch, Vocal abuse, Vocal fold paralysis, Vocal nodule, Vocal polyp

Praxis Area 2: Assessment and Diagnosis

I. Principles of Assessment
  A. List and describe symptoms and causes of vocal pathologies
  B. Identify type and purpose of diagnostic instruments and their purposes

II. Interpretation of Assessment Results
  A. Identify and distinguish disorders of physiological, functional, neurological, and psychological origin
  B. Describe characteristics and match voice quality to etiology

Praxis Area 3: Treatment Planning and Evaluation

I. Principles of Treatment
  A. Recognize need to make referral for medical management
  B. Identify counseling approaches and techniques
  C. Identify risk behaviors of disorders and recommend preventive measures

II. Implementation of Treatment Procedures
  A. Implement treatment approaches and techniques for each disorder type and etiology
  B. Administer training techniques for alaryngeal/esophageal speech

Sample Voice Disorders Question

An adult male has had 3 weeks of voice intervention for contact ulcers but remains dysphonic. The vocal behavior most likely responsible for his lack of progress is:[11]

  A. A speaking fundamental frequency around 125 Hz

B. Beginning voice production with a hard glottal attack

C. Shortened vowel durations in speech

D. Poor velopharyngeal closure

Selecting the correct answer should be quite easy since 3 of the 4 choices, (A), (C), and (D), have no direct effect on voice production. Therefore, (B) is the correct answer. However, abstract reasoning could be used to assist in assessing the effect of each behavior reflected in the choices. Choices (A) and (C) are normal conditions that do not impact progress in voice treatment. Poor velopharyngeal closure has no effect on the ability to phonate, so (D) is incorrect.

Suggested Voice Disorders Resources

Sapienza, C., Hicks, D., & Ruddy, B. (2011). Voice disorders. In N. Anderson & G. Shames (Eds.), *Human communication disorders: An introduction* (pp. 222–253). Boston, MA: Pearson.

Kempster, G. (2015). Voice disorders in children and adults. In G. Lof & A. Johnson (Eds.), *National speech-language pathology examination review and study guide* (pp. 243–262). Evanston, IL: TherapyEd.

Roseberry-McKibbin, C., & Hegde, M. (2018). Voice and its disorders. In *Advanced review of speech-language pathology* (pp. 291–346). Austin, TX: Pro-Ed.

Augmentative and Alternative Communication (AAC)

Praxis Area 1: Foundations

I. Terminology and Concepts
   Aided/Unaided, American Sign Language (ASL), AMER-IND, Blissymbol, Candidacy assessment, Cerebral palsy, Digitized speech, Direct selection, Display, Eye blink encoding, Fitzgerald key system, Iconicity, Iconic symbol, Linear/Row/Column scanning, Low/High technology, Noniconic symbol, Pantomime, Partner-assisted scanning, Pic symbol, Picture Exchange Communication System (PECS), Premack symbol, Rate enhancement, Rebus, Scanning pattern, Sig symbol, Speech generating device, Symbol transparency, Synthesized speech, Switch, Text-to-speech, Visual scanning

Praxis Area 2: Assessment and Diagnosis

I. Principles of Assessment
   A. Identify and distinguish types of AAC systems
   B. Identify properties and pros and cons of various AAC systems
   C. Identify and distinguish symbols systems

II. Implementation of Assessment Protocols
   A. Assess candidacy for temporary or permanent AAC system
   B. Assess need for use of direct selection or scanning

Praxis Area 3: Treatment Planning and Evaluation

I. Treatment Principles
   A. Distinguish low- and high-technology systems and make appropriate recommendations based on the client's needs and skills
   B. Match etiology, residual skills, and communication needs to type of AAC system
   C. Train partners and facilitators
   D. Work collaboratively with other professionals

Sample AAC Question

Which of the following is a reasonable intervention strategy for maintaining communication in a client with advanced amyotrophic lateral sclerosis (ALS)?[12]

   A. Raising vocal pitch

   B. Prescribing an electrolarynx

   C. Teaching diaphragmatic breathing

   D. Providing an appropriate augmentative system

Critiquing is the reasoning skill most useful for this question. ALS is a progressive, degenerative neuromuscular disease in which the nerves lose the ability to enervate muscles, even though language remains intact. Critiquing each of the choices, (A), (B), and (C) should be eliminated since these strategies would not results in sustained outcomes. Therefore, (D) is the correct answer.

Suggested AAC Study Resources

Kangas, K., & Lloyd, L. (2011). Augmentative and alternative communication. In N. Anderson & G. Shames (Eds.), *Human communication disorders: An introduction*(pp. 436–470). Boston, MA: Pearson.

Gutmann, M. (2015). Augmentative and alternative communication. In G. Lof & A. Johnson (Eds.), *National speech-language pathology examination review and study guide* (pp. 393–408). Evanston, IL: TherapyEd.

Roseberry-McKibbin, C., & Hegde, M. (2018). Language disorders in children. In *Advanced review of speech-language pathology* (pp. 105–148). Austin, TX: Pro-Ed.

Neurogenic Language Disorders

Praxis Area 1: Foundations

I. Terminology and Concepts
   Alzheimer's disease, Angular gyrus, Anomic aphasia, Auditory comprehension, Auditory/Verbal agnosia, Basal ganglia, Broca's area/aphasia, Circumlocution, Conduction aphasia, Confabulation, Functional communication, Global aphasia, Hemiparesis, Hippocampus, Huntington's disease, Left side neglect, Melodic Intonation Therapy (MIT), Middle cerebral artery, Mini Mental State Examination, Neologism, Oral apraxia, Paralysis, Paraphasic speech, Paresis, Parkinson's disease, Pick's disease, Prognosis, Right hemisphere syndrome, Spontaneous recovery, Subcortical aphasia, Thalamus, Transcortical sensory/ motor aphasia, Visual/Tactile agnosia, Wernicke's area/aphasia, Word naming

Praxis Area 2: Assessment and Diagnosis

I. Determination of Etiology
   A. Identify and distinguish types of aphasia
   B. Relate neuroanatomical structures to functions and types of aphasia
   C. Relate each type of aphasia to locus of lesion and speech and language characteristics
   D. Predict type of aphasia and speech and language characteristics from site of lesion

II. Implementation of Assessment Procedures
   A. Distinguish neurogenic language disorders from neuromotor speech disorders
   B. Recognize right hemisphere disorder and its symptoms
   C. Identify neurodegenerative syndromes and distinguish from aphasia
   D. Identify standardized language assessments and their purposes
   E. Administer and interpret results of diagnostic tests

Praxis Area 3: Treatment Planning and Evaluation

I. Treatment Principles
   A. List and describe treatment approaches
   B. Identify and define treatment programs and their purpose
   C. Identify techniques for treatment of specific deficits
   D. Match type of aphasia to treatment program
   E. Identify factors influencing prognosis for recovery

II. **Implementation of Treatment Procedures**
   A. Select intervention targets based on speech and language characteristics
   B. Construct and prioritize objectives based on clients' needs and abilities
   C. Implement steps of various treatment programs

Sample Neurogenic Language Disorders Question

Since confrontation-naming difficulties are known to be an enduring deficit of most aphasia syndromes, the speech-language pathologist can best help a client with acute aphasia by doing which of the following?[13]

   A. Testing naming by using only pictures or objects as stimuli
   B. Implementing a treatment plan that focuses on improving the naming of pictures
   C. Implementing a treatment plan that focuses on improving the naming of objects
   D. Implementing a treatment plan that focuses on creating or encouraging alternative or compensatory strategies

Several test-taking strategies and the reasoning skill of predicting the examiner will assist in selecting the correct answer. Using the test-taking strategy of avoiding extremes, (A) should be eliminated, while avoiding opposites will lead to elimination of (B) and (C). The reasoning skill of predicting the examiner will lead to selection of the correct answer, (D), since it is the most socially acceptable and reasonable action.

Suggested Neurogenic Language Disorders Study Resources

Holland, A. (2011). Aphasia and related acquired language disorders. In N. Anderson & G. Shames (Eds.), *Human communication disorders: An introduction* (pp. 409–435). Boston, MA: Pearson.

Nicholas, M. (2015). Acquired language disorders: Aphasia, right-hemisphere disorders and neurogenerative syndromes. In G. Lof & A. Johnson (Eds.), *National speech-language pathology examination review and study guide* (pp. 255–298). Evanston, IL: TherapyEd.

Roseberry-McKibbin, C., & Hegde, M. (2018). Neurologically based communicative disorders and dysphagia. In *Advanced review of speech-language pathology* (pp. 347–414). Austin, TX: Pro-Ed.

Swallowing Disorders

Praxis Area 1: Foundations

I. Terminology and Concepts

Aspiration pneumonia, Bedside evaluation, Buccinators, Chin tuck, Cranial nerves, Cricopharyngeus, Effortful swallow, Electromyography, Electrostimulation, Endoscopy, Epiglottis, Esophageal phase, Esophagostomy, Faucial pillars, Fiberoptic endoscopic evaluation, Gastroscopy, Laryngoscopy, Mandible, Manometry, Mastication, Maxilla, Mendelsohn maneuver, Modified barium swallow, Multiple sclerosis, Muscles of swallowing, Myasthenia gravis, Nasogastric feeding, Oral phase, Oral preparatory phase, Penetration, Peristalsis, Pharyngeal-esophageal sphincter, Pharyngeal phase, Pharyngostomy, Postural techniques, Reflux, Scintigraphy, Supraglottic swallow, Thermal/Tactile stimulation, Tongue thrust, Ultrasound, Velleculae, Velopharyngeal closure, Wallenberg's syndrome

II. **Normal Swallow**
  A. Identify anatomical structures and functions and describe swallow physiology
  B. Identify and describe phases of the swallow process
  C. Identify the purpose of swallowing treatment
  D. Identify causes of swallowing disorders and their effects

Praxis Area 2: Assessment and Diagnosis

I. **Implementation and Interpretation of Assessment Procedures**
  A. Identify and describe activities of the bedside swallow evaluation
  B. Identify and contrast instruments and procedures and their purposes for swallowing evaluation
  C. Interpret results and findings of instrumental evaluation

Praxis Area 3: Treatment Planning and Evaluation

I. **Implementation of Treatment Procedures**
  A. Identify and distinguish direct and indirect treatments and their purposes
  B. Match treatment strategies to specific needs of the client
  C. Recommend specific diet modifications according to needs of the client
  D. Interpret videographic and radiologic images
  E. Recommend techniques for prevention of aspiration

Sample Swallowing Disorders Question

A clinician who wants to examine the oral preparatory, oral, pharyngeal, and cervical stages of a patient's swallowing would most appropriately choose which of the following procedures?[14]

  A. Ultrasonography
  B. Videofluoroscopy

C. Fiberoptic endoscopic evaluation

D. Electromyography

Although the question requires verbatim recall, the reasoning skill of comparison should lead you to the correct answer, (B). Since the question relates to observation of the bolus in each swallowing phase continuously and sequentially, the only procedure that allows this is videofluoroscopy. The other choices, (A), (C), and (D), might assess each phase singularly, so they are incorrect.

Suggested Swallowing Disorders Study Resources

Sonies, B. (2011). Swallowing: process and disorders. In N. Anderson & G. Shames (Eds.), *Human communication disorders: An introduction* (pp. 471–503). Boston, MA: Pearson.

Sonies, B. (2015). Dysphagia: Swallowing and swallowing disorders. In G. Lof & A. Johnson (Eds.), *National speech-language pathology examination review and study guide* (pp. 363–392). Evanston, IL: TherapyEd.

Roseberry-McKibbin, C., & Hegde, M. (2018). Neurologically based communicative disorders and dysphagia. In *Advanced review of speech-language pathology* (pp. 347–414). Austin, TX: Pro-Ed.

Motor Speech Disorders

Praxis Area 1: Foundations

I. **Terminology and Concepts**

Agrammatism, Amyotrophic lateral sclerosis, Apraxia, Apraxia profile, Ataxic dysarthria, Athetosis, Broca's area, Bulbar palsy, Cerebral palsy, Childhood apraxia, Chorea, Diadochokinesis, Delayed auditory feedback, Dysarthria, Dystonia, Extrapyramidal system, Flaccid dysarthria, Guillain-Barré syndrome, Huntington's disease, Hypo/Hyperkinetic dysarthria, Kaufman Speech Praxis Test, Lower/Upper motor neuron, Metastatic error, Mixed dysarthrias, Moebius syndrome, Muscular incoordination, Myoclonus, Nonverbal oral apraxia, Pitch break, Positioning error, Prolongation, Prosody, Rigidity, Screening Test for Developmental Apraxia of Speech, Spasm, Spastic dysarthria, Spasticity, Verbal Motor Production Assessment for children, Visi pitch, Wilson's disease

Praxis Area 2: Assessment and Diagnosis

I. **Etiology and Diagnostic Principles**

A. Identify, differentiate, and classify types of motor speech disorders

B. Relate neuroanatomical structures and locus of lesion to types of motor speech disorders

C. Identify neurodegenerative syndromes

D. Predict type of motor speech disorder from site of lesion

E. Distinguish motor speech disorders from neurogenic language disorders

II. **Implementation of Assessment Procedures**

A. Identify standardized assessments and their purposes

B. Interpret test results and classify severity

C. Recognize and classify prognostic indicators; formulate a prognosis

Praxis Area 3: Treatment Planning and Evaluation

I. **Treatment Principles**

A. Identify and describe treatment approaches and their purposes

B. Match treatment strategies to specific disorders and individual needs of the client

II. **Implementation of Treatment Procedures**

A. Select and prioritize treatment goals

B. Select treatment targets and stimuli

C. Utilize performance data to determine next step or terminate treatment

D. Recommend augmentative and alternative communication systems and match features to clients' needs, abilities, and prognosis

Sample Motor Speech Disorders Question

Which of the following sets of speech characteristics is most likely to be exhibited by an individual with ataxic dysarthria?[15]

A. Monopitch, reduced stress, rapid alternative motion rates, short rushes of speech, and increased rate within segments of connected speech

B. Short rushes of speech, hypernasality, pitch breaks, inhalatory stridor, and rapid alternative motion rates

C. Low voice pitch, strained-strangled voice quality, pitch breaks, harshness, and slow but regular alternating motion rates

D. Irregular articulatory breakdowns, excess and equal stress, prolonged phonemes, irregular alternating motion rates, and slow rate of connected speech

This question may require additional time since the correct answer is not immediately apparent and each answer choice contains several elements. Since ataxic dysarthria is the result of a lesion to the cerebellum, the reasoning skills of critiquing and abstract reasoning should be utilized as you consider each element with the answer choices as related to ataxic dysarthria. Thus, ataxic dysarthria would produce motoric problems in coordination of the articulatory muscles. Using critiquing, (A), (B), and (C) should be eliminated because they contain elements related to voice production. Using abstract reasoning, muscular incoordination problems are most appropriately described by (D), so this is the correct answer.

Suggested Motor Speech Disorders Study Resources

Freed, D. (2020). *Motor speech disorders: Diagnosis and treatment.* San Diego, CA: Plural Publishing.

Murdoch, B. (2011). Neurogenic disorders of speech in children and adults. In N. Anderson & G. Shames (Eds.), *Human communication disorders: An introduction.* San Diego, CA: Pearson.

Turner, G. (2015). Motor Speech Disorders. In G. Lof & A. Johnson (Eds.), *National speech-language pathology examination review and study guide* (pp. 299–330). Evanston, IL: TherapyEd.

Roseberry-McKibbin, C., & Hegde, M. (2018). Neurologically based communicative disorders and dysphagia. In *Advanced review of speech-language pathology* (pp. 347–414). Austin, TX: Pro-Ed.

Traumatic Brain Injury

Praxis Area 1: Foundations

I. **Terminology and Concepts**
Acceleration injury, Amnesia, Behavior disorders, Brief Test of Head Injury, Cognitive assessment, Closed/Open head injury, Cognitive disorders, Concussion, Confabulation, Confrontation naming, Disability rating scale, Discourse deficit, Dysphagia, Executive function, Family members, Glasgow Coma Scale, Language disorders, Motor speech disorders, Neuroplasticity, Nonacceleration injury, Perseveration, Pragmatic language disorder, Problem solving, Rancho Los Amigos Levels of Cognitive Function, Reintegration, Social functioning

Praxis Area 2: Assessment and Diagnosis

I. **Assessment Principles**
   A. Identify and describe characteristics of speech/language and cognitive function
   B. Identify purpose for assessment, select appropriate procedures/instruments, and interpret results

II. **Implementation of Assessment Procedures**
   A. Identify standardized assessment tools and their purposes
   B. Administer test instruments and interpret their results

   C. Recognize and classify prognostic indicators; formulate a prognosis

   D. Recognize defense mechanisms and need for counseling

Praxis Area 3: Treatment Planning and Evaluation

  I. Implementation of Treatment

    A. Identify appropriate treatment for disorder characteristics and severity

    B. Match intervention strategies to specific needs of the client

    C. Determine most effective strategy to elicit and maintain desired behavior

    D. Prioritize steps in the treatment process

    E. Utilize performance data to determine next step or terminate treatment

    F. Identify and implement appropriate behavior management techniques

    G. Recognize client counseling approaches and techniques

    H. Implement counseling techniques

Sample Traumatic Brain Injury Question

Head trauma resulting from motor vehicle accidents, falls, or sports injuries often leads to changes in a child's cognitive functioning that can affect behavior and learning patterns. Which of the following is the most appropriate strategy for the speech-language pathologist in beginning to work with a child who has suffered a head trauma?[16]

    A. Rekindle the child's premorbid concept of being normal before initiating specific speech and language intervention.

    B. Begin with rote language tasks with high levels of success before progressing to tasks that are more challenging.

    C. Begin with elicitation of complex linguistic structures and regress to simpler linguistic material if the child is unable to perform complex tasks.

    D. Strengthen the child's motor skills before implementing specific speech and language intervention activities.

Questions involving clinical decision making always initially require the reasoning skill of comparison to rule out untenable choices. Use of comparison should immediately lead to elimination of (A) and (D) since the actions are not typically in the practice domain of speech-language pathology. The remaining choices, (B) and (C), appear to be opposites; however, use of the reasoning skill of predicting the examiner should lead to elimination of (C) since it is not reasonable to expose a child to frustration and failure. Therefore, the correct answer is (B).

Suggested Traumatic Brain Injury Study Resources

Weismer, G., & Brown, D. (2019). *Introduction to communication sciences and disorders: The scientific basis of clinical practice.* San Diego, CA: Plural Publishing.

Roseberry-McKibbin, C., & Hegde, M. (2018). Neurologically based communicative disorders and dysphagia. In *Advanced review of speech-language pathology* (pp. 347–414). Austin, TX: Pro-Ed.

Research Methods

Praxis Area 1: Foundations

I. **Terminology and Concepts**
ABA/ABAB design, Case study, Cause/Effect, Correlation, Cross-sectional study, Descriptive research, Developmental research, Experimental/Control groups, Experimental research, Ex post facto, Generalization, Hypothesis, Independent/Dependent variables, Interval data/scale, Longitudinal study, Mean/Mode/Median, Normative study, Null hypothesis, Ordinal data/scale, Pre/Post-test, Qualitative data/research, Quantitative data/research, Randomization, Range, Reliability, Research hypothesis, Significant difference, Single-case design, Standard deviation, Time-series design, Validity, Variable

II. **Types of Data, Research Designs, and Their Uses**
   A. Distinguish types of research designs
   B. Identify types of data and variables
   C. Identify and construct hypotheses
   D. Recognize measures of central tendency, validity, and reliability
   E. Critique research studies for reliability and validity
   F. Draw appropriate conclusions from research findings

Praxis Area 2: Assessment and Diagnosis

I. **Evidence-Based Assessment Practice**
   A. Apply psychometric and statistical concepts to assessment
   B. Administer test items with reliability
   C. Select valid test instruments
   D. Interpret test scores using norm, percentile, age equivalency, stanine, quartile
   E. Categorize severity of a disorder based on test score

Praxis Area 3: Treatment Planning and Evaluation

I. **Evidence-Based Treatment Practices**
   A. Utilize data to measure and document performance outcomes
   B. Use appropriate data for SOAP notes
   C. Plan treatment strategies based on research findings
   D. Evaluate and document treatment efficacy

Sample Research Methods Question

A study of the effect of a drug on stuttering involved administering the drug to one group of 20 people who stutter and a placebo to another group of 20 people who stutter. The groups were matched in age, gender, and severity of stuttering. Amount of stuttering was measured before and after the experimental procedure. In this experiment, which of the following is the dependent variable?[17]

    A. Amount of stuttering

    B. The drug

    C. Age

    D. Gender

After eliminating (C) and (D) since they are the matching criteria for the two groups, if you have difficulty distinguishing between the dependent and independent variable in a research study, you should utilize the reasoning skill of cluing. Using cluing, the dependent variable refers to the variable that is measured. Since the question contains the phrase "Amount of stuttering was measured," (A) would be a good choice and the correct answer.

Suggested Research Methods Study Resources

Hegde, M., & Salvatore, A. (2020). *Clinical research in communication disorders: Principles and strategies.* San Diego, CA: Plural Publishing.

Greenwald, M. (2015). Research, evidence-based practice and tests and measurements. In G. Lof & A. Johnson (Eds.), *National speech-language pathology examination review and study guide* (pp. 91–102). Evanston, IL: TherapyEd.

Roseberry-McKibbin, C., & Hegde, M. (2018). Research design and statistics: A foundation for clinical science. In *Advanced review of speech-language pathology* (pp. 563–600). Austin, TX: Pro-Ed.

Multicultural Issues

Praxis Area 1: Foundations

  I. **Terminology and Concepts**

      Alternatives to standardized tests, Bilingual education, Code switching, Criterion-referenced test, Dialect, Difference versus disorder, Disproportionality, Dominant language, Dynamic assessment, English as a Second Language (ESL), Health disparity, Interpreters, Native language, Risk factors, Second language acquisition characteristics, Test bias/modification, Test translation

  II. **Disability and Education Law**

      A. Individuals With Disabilities Education Act (IDEA)

    B. Americans With Disabilities Act (ADA)

    C. Bilingual Education Act

III. **Major Multicultural Populations: African Americans/Hispanics/Asian Americans/ Pacific Islanders**

    A. Linguistic characteristics

    B. Predispositions to etiological conditions: Social/health/environmental factors

IV. **Bilingualism**

    A. Types of bilingualism

    B. Typical second language acquisition and stages

    C. Characteristics of English Language Learners (ELLs)

Praxis Area 2: Assessment and Diagnosis

I. **Culturally Sensitive Assessment**

    A. Identify principles of nonbiased assessment

    B. Select and administer culturally appropriate assessment procedures

    C. Interpret test results

    D. Identify alternative assessment procedures

    E. Distinguish normal communication from communication disorders

Praxis Area 3: Treatment Planning and Evaluation

I. **Culturally Sensitive Intervention**

    A. Identify options for placement in bilingual and special education programs

    B. Determine the language for intervention

    C. Identify criteria for use of interpreters

    D. Establish language dominance

    E. Select targets for intervention outcomes

Sample Multicultural Issues Questions

Which of the following is the most appropriate decision for a speech-language pathologist in planning treatment for a 5-year-old ELL child with a language disorder?

    A. The child should receive intervention in English, since English is the language of instruction in the classroom.

    B. The speech-language pathologist should ask the child's parents to select the language for intervention.

    C. The child should receive intervention in the native language since it is the language in the home environment.

    D. After bilingual assessment, intervention should be initiated in the language in which the child is most proficient simultaneously with English if indicated.

Indeed, all of the options are feasible. If you do not recognize the correct answer immediately, you should use the reasoning skills of key words, classification, and values.
The key word, *most appropriate*, is a cue to use your reasoning skill of classification
to arrange the options in hierarchical order. You should also recognize this as a values
question, and thus select the option that reflects the highest standard of the profession.
Hence, the correct answer is (D).

Suggested Multicultural Issues Study Resources

Roseberry-McKibbin, C. (2018). *Multicultural students with special language needs.* Oceanside,
CA: Academic Communication Associates.

Langdon, H., & Saenz, T. (1996). *Language assessment and intervention with multicultural
students.* Oceanside, CA: Academic Communication Associates.

Roseberry-McKibbin, C., & Hegde, M. (2018). Communication disorders in multicultural
populations. In *Advanced review of speech-language pathology* (pp. 414–462). Austin, TX:
Pro-Ed.

Payne, K. (2011). Multicultural and multilingual considerations. In N. Anderson & G. Shames
(Eds.), *Human communication disorders: An introduction* (pp. 93–125). Boston, MA:
Pearson.

References

1. Educational Testing Service. (1995). *A guide to the NTE Speech-Language Pathology Specialty
   Area Test* (p. 63). Princeton, NJ: Author.
2. Ibid. p. 32.
3. Ibid. p. 105.
4. Ibid. p. 89.
5. Ibid. p. 108.
6. Ibid. p. 78.
7. Ibid. p. 81.
8. Ibid. p. 77.
9. Ibid. p. 66.
10. Ibid. p. 91.
11. Ibid. p. 103.
12. Ibid. p. 96.
13. Ibid. p. 72.
14. Ibid. p. 79.
15. Ibid. p. 121.
16. Ibid. p. 110.
17. Ibid. p. 71.

Index